Giggle More, Worry Less:
A Pediatrician's Thoughts for New Parents
By Gregory W. Parkinson, MD, FAAP
Copyright pending 2015

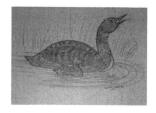

Print Edition
Printed by CreateSpace

Dedicated to my family

A giggle is worth a thousand
worries
Dr P-

Preface

Parents love. Parents worry. Parenthood is a joy. It is difficult and stressful as well. How can you maximize the joy and minimize the stress? That is the goal of this book.

Giggling is perhaps the most beautiful sound in nature. It makes those who hear it smile, especially when it comes from a child. Doctors' offices have too much crying and not enough giggling. The same is true of many homes.

"Giggle More, Worry Less" is a different kind of parenting book. It is not an encyclopedia. Instead, it focuses on important topics. I want you to understand when to worry, and when to relax. This way you can focus more time on love and having fun- giggling, as it were.

Common sense is central to my approach, and so is compassion and so is a sense of humor. You will learn "How to manipulate your mother" and that "Spit happens". Each of the topics is covered in just a few pages, so you can choose what you need, when you need it.

As a pediatrician and father for 20 years, I have learned to laugh at myself and to adapt. My approach to pediatrics is traditional. Having said that, I am willing to question whether our teaching makes sense. With experience, you learn that even absolute, official guidelines have a habit of evolving every few years. Just ask your parents- they will tell you that "everything has changed" since you were a baby.

Learning to listen is essential. Patients and parents are often trying to tell the doctor what is going on if he or she is just able to listen. The same is true for babies communicating with their parents.

This book ultimately tries to hone in on things that every parent should know. If I could sit down and share with you, this is what I would share.

I hope it helps.

Chapters:

A note about gender-specific pronouns (he and she, that is)

Throughout this book, there are many specific times when I refer to your baby (or occasionally to your doctor). Rather than awkwardly say *he/she* every time, most chapters pick one gender or the other. You should not make any value judgment on the gender chosen. In general, I have alternated chapters. Exceptions occur when it is appropriate (the circumcision chapter, for example, refers to *he*).

Chapter 1: Introduction

a. Children keep you young, but first they make you old.

I saw this on a postcard once. We kept it posted at the office. Truer words were never spoken. This applies to anyone that works or interacts with kids, but is especially the case for parents. The stress of parenting is not something you can really *get* until you live it. Becoming a parent is like opening a door to a room you barely knew existed.

It begins during pregnancy, and then escalates at birth, when you realize that the little creature in the bassinet is totally dependent on you. Perhaps women realize this sooner than men. As one buddy of mine said before his first child's birth, "How hard can it be? They sleep, they eat and they poop." His co-workers (who were already parents or grandparents) just smiled. A week after his son's birth, as he arrived bleary-eyed to his office, an explanation of how hard it can be no longer seemed necessary. This is how parenthood begins: feeding and bouncing and rocking and singing. It is amazing how staying up all night with someone will bond you to him (it's true for doctors and patients, too.)

Certain situations will sharply accelerate the aging. I refer to these as *your future gray hairs*. Mine are evenly divided among experiences with my own family and my patients. It could be his first fever, her first fall, the time she figures out the child safety lock or when he cries the first day at preschool.... you get the idea. These will seem small in comparison when the teen years arrive. Little kids, little problems; big kids, big problems, as they say. But if you're just starting out, you don't want to hear that yet. The truth may be that the current problem often seems the most pressing. The elderly will tell you that it doesn't stop when your children reach adulthood either.

At the same time, these seniors will also demonstrate how a child can ward off aging. Just watch a grandmother playing kickball, a grandfather pushing a stroller or an older teacher trying to learn this year's high school slang. Pediatricians get the benefit of this every day, and I think most of us would take this any day over a wrinkle cream.

So if your father was like mine and said to you, "Hardest job you'll ever have, being a parent, you know", you'll probably agree sooner or later. Hopefully you'll think it' s the best job, too.

b. You don't need to know everything- just listen

As new parents, you make a lot of decisions. At times, it will seem overwhelming to choose wisely for your family. To make matters worse, everyone will have an opinion about raising your child- friends, family, magazines, the Internet, doctors, nurses and sometimes even complete strangers in the grocery checkout line! How can you make sense of all this advice?

Parenting is a journey. You are travelling on *the road of life*. You are your child's driver: you are part chauffeur, part tour guide, and part chaperone. As with any trip, the people taking it are the ones that matter. This begins with your baby. A smart mother will listen to her baby. Although there is a lot of anxiety in making decisions, it is not as complicated as you might think. You really just want her to be safe, happy, healthy and well adjusted. If you listen to her when choosing your route, you will make decisions that lead you in the right direction.

By listening to your baby and to one another, you will develop an internal compass. Let's look at the example of when your baby cries. She can't verbalize what she wants, but you will have an idea that she *needs* something. You pick her up, hold her, bounce her, feed her or change her until you find what stops the crying. When she stops crying, she is telling you that you figured it out. You have listened and learned. With time, you will see patterns and develop an intuition about what she needs: crying after a long sleep

8

probably means she is hungry, while crying after a good feed means she needs to burp. By learning your baby's needs, you will help direct your actions in more ways than you realize. For instance, if your baby doesn't cry in the evening, you might feel good about trying to take her on an outing, whereas if this is her fussy time, you probably will have her stay home.

Be patient with yourself in this process. Learning takes time. Many new parents have the right instincts, but lack confidence. This is natural, especially when you have a crying baby in front of you! Stay calm, stick with your plan and you will usually get there. Staying calm will help your baby as well.

Listening also helps when you are looking at bigger issues, like where to live, whether or not to work outside the home and so on. Trust your gut. This seems very basic, but it is really important. When you are comfortable, not only are you more likely to make a better choice, you will have less stress and more confidence. This builds on itself over time and makes you a better and happier parent.

Trusting your gut is looking inward, or *internalizing* a decision. This is as opposed to letting outside influences like the Internet guide you, which is *externalizing* the decision. When externalizing, you lose control and forfeit your judgment at the same time. When you will get conflicting advice from different sources, your head ends up spinning. It will be harder to choose well and you will suffer in confidence and parenting ability. When you trust yourself, you will be right more often. Even when you are wrong, there is still a feeling of comfort in the way you made the decision. On the other hand, when you don't trust yourself and it turns out badly, you kick yourself for a long time.

In a two-parent relationship, your partner will be going through the same process of listening and learning. In strong relationships, decisions can be discussed and (usually) agreed upon. You navigate together. This has multiple benefits: you are each other's sounding board, confidant and partner. Of course, sometimes you will both listen, but *hear* differently. This will require negotiation. Overall, though, you will not only help your child, but also strengthen your own bond.

You are embarking on a challenging, stressful, exciting and joyous journey. You will learn a lot along the way. Rest assured that for most decisions, both big and small, there are several paths you can take. Listen to your baby, your partner and yourself. Then, choose the route that you think will make you and your child happy. This simple plan will help to make your journey a pleasant one.

c.   Four helpers- for what you don't know

A good doctor *knows what she doesn't know*, and knows when to ask for help. The same is true of good parents. Most new parents will need a lot of help. Although your baby, your partner and you are steering your course, a good pit crew makes it easier to stay on track. I recommend a four-piece crew: one family member, one friend, one medical caregiver and one book or website. This will give you a cross section of those that know you and your baby, and those that know about children. It will also avoid information overload.

The most common family member is consult is one of the grandmothers. A grandmother has both the experience and the motivation to give good advice. Every emergency room could reduce their wait times and costs with a good grandmother out front, deciding who should go home and who needs to be see the doctor. If you are lucky, relying on your own mother or mother-in-law will bring you closer, and will give you a new sense of appreciation and respect for her.

Not everyone is lucky. Sometimes a grandmother is deceased or unavailable. And sometimes she is downright negative. In that case, you have probably already thought of another person to whom you can turn. If you choose a confidante who is not a family elder, it may well ruffle some feathers. Consider this in your decision, especially if you live with extended family. Also think about who will be caring for the baby if you are at work. Providing child-care often makes a relative feel empowered to offer opinions. Ultimately, though, you get the final say. Make a careful decision and stand by it.

Friends are great because we get to choose them. Good qualities in advisor/friends can include a medical background, experience as a parent (especially if you like how her kids are turning out) or just a good shoulder on which to lean or cry. Choosing this person gives the most flexibility, and you can pick a person whose qualities are not present in your other resource people.

Nine months of pregnancy gives you a lot of time to pick your crew. It is like a long tryout. And you may be surprised by how some of the players respond, both for better and for worse. This is especially true of friends. Pregnancy is obviously a huge transition in a person's life. Not quite so obvious is how this transition brings you closer to some friends and distances you from others. Some people are great at socializing but are not great at sitting with you on bed-rest or at playtime. Others step up and step in. The situation tends to clarify itself if you are looking for the signs.

Some people don't quite make the cut as advisors. Since you don't actually say, "I'm choosing to not listen to you", don't expect the unsolicited advice to go away. In fact, those whose advice you least want tend to be more forward about offering it. Learning to say, "Oh thank you, I'll have to do that" can be very useful and non-confrontational, even if you have no intention of listening. It also allows you to take advantage of the rare times that you are offered something helpful.

We will talk later about how to choose a pediatrician/other medical provider, but clearly this person is your main source for medical information. A good provider will provide you with options for most decisions, with the pros and cons of each so you can decide. She will occasionally need to be firm when there is one clear best decision in a situation. Personally, I try to be the AAA guy. I tell you about the main road and the side roads on your trip and will try to guide you either way you prefer. Occasionally, though, if you are travelling on the wrong side of the road or in the wrong direction, I will clearly recommend how you should get back on the right route.

The Internet has brought information overload and anxiety to a whole new level for today's parents. You will be shocked at the differences in opinion even between experts. This is because there is more than one good way to tackle most situations. Choose one good website or book that can answer most of your questions. There is no better place to start than the American Academy of Pediatrics website, http://www.aap.org, or alternately the AAP's well child book, Caring for You Baby and Young Child.

Clearly, this is just a guide; the idea is for you to have a framework of support. There will be situations when your regular resources are not the right ones. You can certainly have substitutes for particular needs. For example, if your baby is colicky, perhaps your aunt who went through the same thing can help more than your mother. If you are breastfeeding, the lactation consultant might substitute for the doctor. If your child needs to see a specialist, she can take the place of your primary care provider. And a specific web site may be great for a particular issue, such as the Center for Disease Control (www.cdc.gov) or Children's Hospital of Philadelphia (http://www.chop.edu/service/vaccine-education-center) for immunization information.

With your team in place, you will be well prepared for the adventures that follow. No one has a crystal ball to predict where the road will lead, but good people and good information will help to point you in the right direction.

d.   There should be a Purple Heart for parenthood.

I have an immense respect for parents. It is an entirely earned respect, from years of observation. Pediatricians see it from the moment of birth. Right after delivery, after a new mother's *Thank God that's over* feelings pass, when she holds her child for the first time, her expression changes to what can only be described as *Wow!* She realizes that she and the father made that little person. It is quite remarkable.

Shortly thereafter, most new mothers will have a moment when the penny seems to drop. At this instant, there is a realization of the worry that comes with parenthood. Although pregnancy itself begins this thought process, seeing the baby puts it into full effect.

Some will even say, "Now, I know why my mother worries so much!"

Childbirth gives a woman more than just a new appreciation of her own mother. It teaches her what all mothers learn-that the two essences of being a mother are responsibility and love. Responsibility is an absolute and unequivocal feeling. The two most basic responsibilities are to feed and protect. These seem to be very primitive instincts. I'm not sure if birds love their babies, but they still feed and protect them.   These actions are so important that they have been maintained up through evolution (1).

Knowing that responsibility is a primitive instinct makes it easier for me to understand why mothers worry so much. It is nature's way of making sure nothing bad happens- if a mother worries about everything, then nothing will get missed. The more evolved part of our human brain can *override* the feeling of worry and reassure itself – this is especially true with experience. For example, if a second–time parent drops a pacifier on the floor, she might invoke the *five-second rule*, when the thought of this would have been horrifying with the first child.

Love is, of course, much more complicated. I won't even attempt to get my head around it, expect to draw a distinction between loving your child, and being *in love* with him. Almost all mothers love their children, meaning that it gives the mother pleasure to see the children healthy and happy. The lucky mothers are also in love, right from an early age. For these mothers, all the work of caring for a baby can be joyful. Perhaps luck is not the right word, but happiness simply eludes some women for no good reason. It is tremendously difficult for a well-intentioned mother to be depressed. To paraphrase an obstetrician/friend, in describing her own post-partum depression, "The only thing worse than how sad you feel is the guilt that comes when people tell you it should be the happiest moment of your life." Thanks to people like Brooke Shields, post-partum depression is much better accepted than in the past. It is acceptable to talk about for mothers, and increasingly understood by doctors and society. Most importantly, we have moved from blame to sympathy and support. It is seen that mothers show strength by admitting their difficulties, and that courage and dedication are necessary to continue in spite of negative emotions.

Fathers go through their own process, but it has a little more variation. A few guys hover like a second mother. Most think about the traditional role of providing protection, shelter and money. The good ones think about being good dads. Too many men are not involved at all, and some are abusive. New research even suggests some men might go through their own form of post partum depression (2).

There are many men who do step up, and occasionally some who take the lead in the child-rearing role. There are many others who the doctor doesn't see because they are working their butts off to keep the finances afloat. This includes obtaining the all-important health insurance to cover the many medical expenses along the way. And sometimes mothers fail in their duties, for a variety of reasons, and the father does it all.

When a child develops a serious health condition, whether medical, developmental or both, true bravery and dedication become evident. I am repeatedly amazed by parents who forget life as it previously existed, and morph into a combination of nurse, therapist, advocate, rare disease specialist and most of all, foot soldier. Feeding tubes, monitors, syringes and medications become their tools. The duties are undefined and at times there is no relief. Many times I have I thought, "I could not do what you do." All too often, this is the reality for men, as fathers separate themselves, physically, emotionally or both. I have known wives to tell their husbands, "You're either on board with this or you're not, but either way I am going to take care of our child."

There is heroism in many parents, especially mothers, which is badly under-recognized in our society. Inside most women is an almost super-human ability to tolerate adversity for the sake of their children. This receives media attention in extreme circumstances like famine, disaster or war, but seldom in the mundane battle that takes place in homes around the world. It takes incredible strength to care for a disabled child, to get through years of cancer treatment, or to leave everything you own to escape an abusive relationship. The source of this strength is elusive, but it emerges faithfully in times of need. Most mothers will not need to summon it routinely, and they will doubt their ability to do so. Rest assured that, if necessary, it will appear, as it has in so many mothers before.

More fathers need to better understand this part of parenthood. Given the choice between our needs and the needs our children, our children usually win. This is how it should be. By focusing on our kids, men can help in many ways. We can assist our children in what they are going through, we can take a lot of stress off of our partners, and we can bring the family closer together. If you are one of those dads, I salute you, because you are not only doing the right thing, you are setting an example that others can follow. We need more of this kind of courage.

e.   Giggle more

At Falmouth Pediatrics, we work hard. There is a lot of stress in a pediatric office. We also have all kinds of fun. We dress up as an office for Halloween. We play practical jokes and we laugh a lot. Most of all, we love to hear 4 and 5 year olds explain important topics.

Think about your previous experiences at school or work. Which classes did you like? Was there a job you enjoyed? Where did you learn the most? Usually the answer lies in the places where you had fun and found meaning.

We have already talked about the hard work and stress that parenting brings. It is really important to find healthy ways to reduce stress. Having fun and finding humor help. Humor improves coping with stress, and it probably improves how we learn (1). It also helps to keep a positive outlook (2). These are important skills not just for us to acquire, but also for our kids.

My son, Andrew, can make people laugh on demand. His Uncle Mark can tell stories that have us in stitches. Most of us are not so fortunate, but you don't have to be a stand-up comic, nor should you be a full-time entertainer for your child. We all can appreciate fun, though. Fun can be a conscious decision if you make it an option. It is as simple as thinking about what day-to-day activities you and your child enjoy.

For a newborn, fun will simply be what keeps him from crying. After a month or two, first smiles start to make his idea of fun more obvious. If you are fortunate enough to have a belly-laugher, the feedback is almost impossible to resist. Singing a song or reading a story is free and easy. Many kids will spend hours playing peekaboo. These simple activities open entire worlds to young minds- music, literature, and imagination. Outdoors gives the opportunity to stomp in puddles, build sand castles, jump in leaves and make snow angels, depending on the season.

Everyday chores become much less tedious if they are enjoyable. Most babies love their bath. This is great place to teach body parts, and so is the changing table. Folding laundry can help them learn to match things. Even in the kitchen, we used to put fridge letters in a big pot on the floor – stir it up with a spoon and you've got alphabet soup!

Once they start talking, kids truly will start entertaining you by accident with their words and actions. When he calls a backpack a 'packpack', you may have to hide your smirking from him, but you will have a great memory for yourself. Cherish words like 'lellow' (for yellow) as long as they last. When they are older, kids always want to know what funny things they used to say.

Finally, and may be most importantly, laughing is probably the best cure I know for sadness. We have all had the experience of laughing so hard we cry, or crying to the point where we start to laugh. Some days you will be exhausted. The baby will be fussy, and just when you get her down, the dog will start barking. Being able to step back and see humor in a lousy situation is a huge help.

It also shows that we don't take ourselves too seriously. When you're a parent, that can be the biggest joke of all.

f. Older parents never regret spending too much time with their children.

Time is our most precious commodity. Plentiful at birth, it slowly slips away like sand through an hourglass. Not knowing exactly how much we own, we must still try to distribute it wisely. Although this represents one of life's greatest and most important challenges, how much conscious thought do we give it?

We can overcome the immensity of this question by thinking about it just for one day. What is the best use of your time today? From there, you can extend it to a typical day. In concrete terms, we hope to spend about eight hours sleeping. The second eight hours (at least) will probably be occupied by our main duties, whether that is childcare or working outside the home. If we are lucky, the remaining third of the day has some degree of flexibility, and may allow us some control. On the small scale, this is a good place to focus. I can't imagine really having a full eight hours of free time, nor does it seem like a good idea to over-schedule that time. Still, a little thought about how to allocate commuting, chores, and activities will go a long way.

Medical school actually provides a great education in time management. First of all, you are so darned busy with studying and clinical work. Second, any free time you get tends to be on off hours, so that getting a haircut or going to a bank poses a major challenge. In this way, parenthood is very similar- lots to do, and very little time in which to do it.

Observing the time allocation of my medical mentors was one of the most important parts of my education, even though I seldom discussed the mental notes being made. Over time it became clear that life's commitments are like a triangle – with the three corners represented by family life, work life and personal interests. Doctors are frequently workaholics, and many are only really good at work. Many of my supervising doctors did a very good job at two out of three, but no one could realistically excel at all three. Twenty-five years later, that still seems about right.

I decided that if grades were being handed out, my goal would be to get an A on my family and an A on my patients. The personal corner - fitness, hobbies etc.- was important, but it would be the one that would have to give at times. Maybe a C+ would be realistic. This certainly is not very glamorous. In fact, my teenagers would call my life downright boring. If Sandee and I succeeded, maybe the kids will thank us later.

You can make your own goals as you see fit. Your life situations will greatly affect your time decisions. Do you have a partner? Do family or friends take an active role with your children? How much do the adults need to work? These are all important questions.

Your first days of parenthood will be filled with simply trying to figure out the baby's sleeping, eating, diaper changes and fussy times. You probably won't be able to imagine time for anything else. Most new parents spend a lot of time in pajamas, and struggle to fit a shower into the day. Within a month or two, a routine will emerge and a few small windows of *non-baby time* will open.

For most families, the first major adjustment is a return to work or school for one or both parents. In the ideal world, everyone would work enough to get personal fulfillment, and a bit of grown-up time, without taking away from the baby. This might exist on some planet, but in 21st century America it is pretty rare. We all struggle with bills and bosses, commuting and so on. Every family has to negotiate a compromise that will help it to be happy, healthy and financially stable. The right answer is different for everyone. Sometimes we have to accept short-term hardship to complete an education that will allow for a better life. Other times, there is no end in sight to two jobs and overtime just to make ends meet. Many families have one parent deployed in the military. These are difficult struggles, but certainly there is a silver lining when children later realize the sacrifice that was made on their behalf.

Most of us, fortunately, have some degree of choice in the amount of time that we spend with our children. Should I stay at home, work-part-time or full time? Should I go for the promotion, or endure the longer commute? Am I going to join that committee, team or club? These are really hard decisions, and no one correct answer exists. The point is to realize that there are only twenty-four hours in the day. Whenever we add time to something outside of family, we take away from time with family. We just need to be thinking about this every day, and *keep our eyes on the prize.*

It came as a great surprise a few years ago when an older physician/colleague expressed regret for working too much during the prime of his career. It left an impression, especially since I have known him to be a very nice guy and an involved grandfather. Many men, especially, seem to realize after the fact that they missed out. I often think about the old Harry Chapin song, "Cats in the Cradle", a father's lament about not being there for his son. I have never heard anyone lament being there too much.

g.   How much space do you take up?

Another great post-card: "If you're not living on the edge, you're taking up too much space." This is easy to understand. Life has a way of becoming very busy. Some of this busy-ness is our own doing. And some of it is imposed on us by society.

Certain things are beyond our control- we all need a home, food and clothing, for example. We have to earn enough money for necessities. Honestly, some of us have more necessities than others. Housing needs to be safe, and is hopefully in a good neighborhood, but *how good* is good, and *how big* is big enough? The same goes for cars, clothing and electronics. Clearly, these choices affect our bills, which affect our work situations, which affect our free and family time.

Then come the children. Will they go to a daycare, and where? Will we buy books or borrow them from the library? As they get older, you will have to choose schools and extra-curricular activities. Older grandparents may shake their heads at the pace of life that younger generations lead. Granted, it is not as simple anymore as, "Be home by dinner time and don't get into trouble", as it was for my generation.

Consumerism pushes us towards excess. Advertising exists for us to buy more. However, to buy more we need to work more, and to take part in more involved activities takes more time. As I have already said, time is the most precious commodity. A friend of mine was on the pit crew of actor Paul Newman, who apparently was known to say, "I can make more money, but I can't make more time." Time needs to be a conscious part of the decision process, if we want any control over how much space we are taking up.

As always, it is a decision that everyone makes personally. Do you like to keep busy or do you need more downtime? Can I live with one bedroom or do I want four? How much better is the school across town than the one around the corner? In how many activities should I involve my child? Is he going to be groomed for

Harvard, the NFL, or the Julliard? This may sound silly as you start off, but you will meet people who think like this.

It is easy to get caught up doing what everyone else does. Seeing that most people feel overworked and overtired, don't be surprised if you end up that way, too. If you want to end up in a better place, you have to think about where it is and how to get there. You need to know where you are going to get where you want to go.

h. Five keys to a child's health

There are really only about five things that are necessary for a child to be healthy. This may seem too few to be true, but I firmly believe it.

First on the list is safety. Safety begins at birth with safe sleep, safe feeding and prevention of falls. Beginning at about 4 months, the perils that result from moving around arrive- babies can pick up objects and can choke on what they find, they can grab or knock over things which can result in burns, and they can get access to poisons. And it continues on from there. I do not put safety first lightly, and we will spend several chapters talking about the specifics later on.

Eating healthy, exercise and limits on electronics are lumped together as what you might call lifestyle. Ideal infant nutrition will usually start with breastfeeding. Parents initially model exercise. And if you think it is premature to discuss electronics in infancy, guess again. It is shocking how many kids become regular TV and computer watchers as infants (full disclosure: I do admit to watching *SportsCenter* with one of my babies, but only if he got up for the day at 5:30 am.) Electronics companies continue to heavily market software that will stimulate a baby's brain to learn, but there is no evidence to date that it is beneficial (1).

If your child has a health issue, you need good care, of course. For many conditions, the amount of effort that you put into your child's care really makes a difference. For example, if your child has eczema, moisturizing multiple times daily and avoiding products that irritate the skin takes extra effort, but pay off with healthier skin for your baby. Many doctors will aim for *acceptable* outcomes-you may want to be *exceptional*. These attempts should always be done in consultation your doctor. Trying to do too much can occasionally have risks. Diabetes is an example of a condition where it is really important to control the blood sugar, but trying to run control too tight can result in dangerously low blood sugar. Your care provider can advise you on how to maximize benefits and minimize risks.

A family history of a serious health condition is also very important. Thanks to genetic technology, determination of our future health risks will likely become simple in the not too distant future. For now, the family history is the poor man's genetic test.

Some family medical problems are important to know about early- an increased risk of skin cancer would prompt extra effort in sun protection, for example. As your child ages, more and more issues become relevant.

Last, but certainly not least, is emotional health. I have often said, that for most kids, it is easier to get to age 18 medically healthy than emotionally healthy and safe. If you are safe and happy, you can reach your full potential. If you are not, nothing else really matters. One of the keys to a child's emotional health is the emotional health of her parents, and the reverse is also true. In most families, "if the baby ain't happy, then the momma ain't happy", and as the saying goes, "If Momma ain't happy, ain't nobody happy." Kidding aside, it is essential for parents to try to maximize their own emotional health, if possible, before even thinking about children. Clearly, life doesn't always work that way. Sometimes poor emotional health can lead to decisions that result in pregnancy. Regardless, taking steps to improve your emotional health will pay huge dividends for your child. It will allow you to best focus your time and energy where it belongs: on them.

i.   Stop. Look, then listen- to see if a child is sick

There are a lot of worried parents at a doctor's office - a whole lot of worried parents. No big surprise. As I have said, worry is Mother Nature's way of making sure we are paying attention. You will be the nervous parent of a sick child soon, or maybe have you been already. When this happens, your provider will almost always be less worried than you. This will become apparent from the moment she walks in the exam room. Why is ·this the case? The answer usually comes from the doctor's eyes.

There is a term that doctors use called *gestalt*, which means a pattern that is more than the sum of its parts. For example, let's say your little boy has had a 104-degree fever for three days. Most parents will be very stressed by this. If I enter the room and see him giggling, jumping off a chair or busy playing make-believe, I will be reassured. On the other hand, if she is lying limp in her mother's arms, pale and breathing rapidly, it is an entirely different first impression.

Specifically, there are things for which a doctor looks. We teach medical students that you usually learn more from the doorway than with the stethoscope, because the most important determinants of illness are the big things. We look first for signs like activity level, breathing rate and changes in skin color. As a doctor, you even have to learn to *see* over the telephone. When parents call, three concerning features almost always elicit the answer, "You need to bring your child to the emergency room." The first is rapid, labored breathing. I ask, "Does she look like she just ran (or crawled) the mile?" The next one is dehydration to the point of no urine output. The third is being lethargic, but lethargy requires clarification. Most sick kids are *couch (or lap) potatoes*- they want to lie down or even cuddle with their parents. This can be worrisome to a parent when the child is normally bouncing off the walls. To clarify, I often ask, "If I went to poke your child for a blood test, would she care?" While we don't want to wait until this point, a *"No"* answer to this question is not normal and needs immediate follow-up. In fact, if this is truly the case when you get to the office or emergency room, you can be sure things will start to happen pretty quickly.

The ears add information to the eyes, but this is usually more detail than urgency. For example, even an abnormal heart murmur in a well-looking baby is usually not an emergency, whereas gray or blue color is an emergency, even with no murmur. Wheezing is also important, but not as much as labored breathing. In fact, pediatricians often talk about *happy wheezers-* these are mildly sick kids who might sound loud even to the ear without a stethoscope, but who are smiling and would seem perfectly well if you covered your ears.

There are always exceptions, and common sense should always prevail. For example, a barking cough might sound bad. Throw in stridor (which is the *whoop* sound on breathing in, and which indicates a narrowing of the windpipe) and the concern goes up. Some babies will do this after feeding or when upset, but if every breath is like this, especially all of a sudden, you know there is a problem.

So look first, then listen. This will help you know when to worry a little, and when to worry a lot.

j.   If your gut tells you the doctor is wrong, then listen to your gut

My Dad is 82 years old. He hates hospitals, but I only recently found out why.

As an infant, I developed severe vomiting and became very sick. My parents brought me to the hospital, where I was admitted. After several days, the doctors were still saying that it was a virus. All my parents could see was that I was lethargic, irritable and losing weight. I am guessing that my mother best appreciated the extent of the illness, but it was my dad who made a scene with the nurses, and stormed his way up to the doctor's office. The doctor was apparently warned of my father's impending arrival, and was able to calm him with a promise to personally re-evaluate me. A few hours later, they received a call saying that a blockage had been found, and that telephone consent was needed to perform emergency surgery. I was fine in the end, but poor Dad was never the same in a hospital. The story became legendary in my family.

So, what went wrong with the medical system initially? First of all, doctors tend to think of the most common diagnosis first- for example, a virus. Second, belly-related illnesses are notoriously among the hardest to diagnose. Third, my blockage was intermittent- it would come and go- if it was not present at the moment that the doctors examined me, it would be extremely hard to detect. Doctors put a lot of weight on their eyes, as we previously discussed. If I looked well during the examination (because the problem was intermittent), the seriousness of the condition would be downplayed. Finally, and most importantly, they didn't listen closely enough to my parents.

Doctors know medicine, but parents know their children. Mothers, especially, tend to know every detail of their baby's routine. You will learn your child very quickly, more quickly than you think. When something is out of the ordinary, you will know. At first, you will worry that every problem is serious- experience will help. You will also rely heavily on your healthcare provider. Positive interactions with your provider will build your trust. Good communication will also help. A good doctor will end a sick visit by explaining how the recovery should proceed, as well as when to call for follow-up. For example, poor fluid intake and labored breathing are standard reasons. I often throw in "or no matter what the crazy doctor said, if you are convinced something worse is wrong, then call."

It can be hard to define, but occasionally you get a feeling that something is worse than the doctor makes it out to be. This is your *gut* talking, sending an unspoken signal of fear. In evolution, these feelings help mammals to avoid dangerous situations. They have been honed over thousands of years (1). We all need to listen to our guts. I have to do this when talking to parents on the phone at night. If I hang up, and something does not feel right with the conversation, I call back and change the plan.

You might worry about being placed on some secret list of difficult parents that the provider keeps. I can assure you that being respectful and having some insight into your own anxiety will go a long way. Something like, "I know I am probably just worrying too much, but…" is a good introduction to a clarifying question. Others worry that the doctor will be offended. Honestly, some might, but that is their problem. It is not a parent's job to make my life easy. Instead, your job is to care for and advocate for your child. Parents have flat-out told me that I was not hearing their concerns, and when this happens, they are usually right. We all win when the child gets better.

Challenging the doctor's diagnosis is not something you want to do regularly. In fact, if you repeatedly feel that need, then you probably need to look for a new provider. However, done at the right time, it can make a big difference to your child's health. And if not, at least you will feel better…and that the doctor listened.

Just ask my Dad.

k. Some parents can *feel* when their child is sick

It was my first year as a licensed physician. I was working mainly as a pediatric resident, but did a little moonlighting at a walk-in clinic. A mother brought her son in with a sore throat. His quick strep throat test was negative, so I told her he did not need antibiotics. She insisted that he was acting exactly like the other times when he had strep, and he needed a prescription. I was young and *by the book* enough to not give in. She was adamant I have since come to learn that there are times when this is true- a quick test or culture for strep is negative, but the illness does not get better without antibiotics.

I have thought many times about this encounter over the years. Was I right to go by the book? She was more knowledgeable about her own child, and she may well have been right. Although it was not a serious illness, it taught me an important lesson: parents and caregivers can look at the same child and see two totally different pictures.

A few years later, another mother and child came in. The mother's words still ring clearly. She said, "He looks like he has strep." Did he have a sore throat? No. Fever? No. Positive strep test? He sure did. What began as complete skepticism evolved into deep respect. The child was acting a certain way, the way he did with strep throat, and his mother was in tune with him enough to realize this.

Essentially, a doctor has to rely primarily on objective information-what symptoms and signs are present? How long has there been a fever? Is there a rash, a cough, a headache or a red throat? We have to see or hear the illness. Parents describe the illness, and we listen to their descriptions with varying degrees of ability. The same thing goes for our examination of the child. In contrast, parents are often relying on non-verbal communication from the child; that is, how he acts.

This is especially true on the first day or two of an illness, when many symptoms have yet to develop. Diagnosing the cause of a fever on the first day of illness is like looking down the highway and trying to see what kind of car is coming. It could be a Chevy, but then again, it could be a Ford. With a little more time it will clarify. I can only treat what I see, even though the parent may sense the illness going a different way. This is why parents must feel comfortable calling for follow-up. An illness that seems minor the first day can occasionally turn out to be more serious.

In closing, a few years ago, my own middle child, Andrew, developed strep throat. No fever, no sore throat, just a headache and a belly ache. Strep is well-known to recur. By Andrew's third episode, he said, "Dad, I feel like I have strep throat." He was right, and I had come full circle.

Chapter 2: Preparing the nest

a. Genetic Yahtzee

It is amazing to see which traits your child inherits. My wife, Sandee, and I have been told that my three kids would find each other, even if they were separated at birth. And yet, Andrew looks like me, Christopher looks like Sandee's Dad, and Catherine does not look strikingly like either one of us. But that is only at first glance. With closer inspection, Andrew has Sandee's face shape, Christopher has my face shape, and Catherine has my brother's eyes. And that is just the faces.

You will find the same thing with your children. I call it *genetic Yahtzee*. You probably remember the game where you shake five dice in a cup and try to roll them all the same number. When sperm and egg unite, you have shaken up the genes rather than the dice. And you are dealing with a 100,000 genes, instead of just five dice. Some of the traits are easy to see. We all know who gets Uncle Sal's nose. You can have fun discovering whether the ear lobe is fully attached to the skin or dangles. Is the second toe longer than the first? Is there a cleft in the chin?

With time, personality traits will emerge. If you look closely, these will be evident sooner than you think. An infant can be so social that she will be the life of the party, just like Grandpa. It will seem odd when a child that looks just like one of you, acts like the other. You might think, "Wait a minute. People who look like me don't have belly laughs!" or something similar. Subtle traits will reveal themselves more gradually. She might run fast like her mother or have her father's artistic ability.

Medical conditions can also be inherited. A baby with red hair and fair skin will need to be careful in the sun. Skin rashes and wheezing might be signs of inherited allergies. Of course, many inherited diseases are not initially apparent. Newborn babies are tested for many rare conditions via a small blood sample taken from the baby's heel. The results, which are available within a week or two, allow for early detection of many serious issues. Early detection, in turn, permits earlier treatment, and at times can prevent a health crisis For example, cystic fibrosis is a genetic condition where the mucus of the lung is too thick and food is not digested properly. Early detection prevents malnutrition. In babies whose thyroid gland does not function properly, early treatment helps to preserve brain development. Multiple other problems are less well known, but equally critical to discover before a disaster occurs.

Mothers are tested during pregnancy for a growing number of illnesses. Fathers can then be tested when concerns arise. If a serious condition is present in your family, the best time for testing is before pregnancy, so that you know your risks. The explosion of genetic knowledge has allowed us to learn about new conditions on almost a daily basis. Occasionally, very difficult decisions have to be made about whether to use modern reproductive technologies to avoid conceiving a child with a serious or life-threatening condition.

I sincerely hope that you do not have to contend with any of these issues, and you can spend your time having fun with who looks like whom. Don't be surprised, though, if your child eventually responds to these comments by saying, "I think I look like me!"

b.   On choosing a pediatrician

Choosing a doctor is important, but you might be a little surprised by my view of how to do it.

The qualities of a good physician are straightforward. You want knowledge, judgment, compassion, honesty, technical ability, good communication skills, availability and perhaps punctuality, not necessarily in that order. Actually, that is the key- how should you order these priorities? We would all like the intelligence of Dr. House with the compassion of Mother Teresa, but you live in the real world, and so it is useful to prioritize.

In very rare circumstances, health care issues can determine where you live; for example, if your child has a very rare disease for which the leading authority lives in Chicago or New York. For the rest of us, we live where we live, and have to choose from a fixed number of options. There can be many choices in big cities, or no choices at all in a very small town. Assuming a choice does exist, how do you find the right person?

Good bedside manner is generally the easiest to determine – just ask friends and neighbors who have children. Keep in mind that doctor–family relationships are indeed relationships, so if your friend loves (or hates) Dr. A., it does not guarantee that you will also. However, consistent feedback from several sources will give you confidence. The Internet also abounds with sites that rate providers. Use caution with these sites, as a negative opinion could well come from someone with an ax to grind. Similarly, a practice consultant can *manage* a provider's on-line appearance so that it looks unrealistically positive.

Knowledge and ability are much harder for the average person to determine.

You probably cannot make this assessment alone, but you will know people who can. Ask your obstetrician to whom she brings her children. You might know a local nurse or two, too. I have called emergency departments in other towns for information. ED nurses usually know who is good. Unfortunately, very few community doctors still see their own patients in hospital. Although medical people can be tight-lipped with outsiders about incompetence, when asked specifically who they like, there will likely be knowledge behind the opinion.

Your priorities in a provider will affect your interpretation of what you learn. If extremely premature labor or a need for complicated surgery is an issue, you really are not that worried about bedside manner; you want the person most likely to save your child. Other basic ways to look for competence include seeing if the provider is certified by the American Board of Pediatrics, a member of the American Academy of Pediatrics, and is in good standing with State Medical Board. Similar certifications exist for family practitioners, medicine/pediatrics doctors, nurse practitioners and physician assistants.

Many parents to be opt to interview pediatricians. This is a great idea, although not essential. Many parents come armed with questions recommended by books and web sites. To be honest, most of the questions are not very useful. While it is important to learn whether office hours match your schedule, it is probably better to go to the practice web site or call the office manager. The interview is more of a first date. What is said is less important than how you feel when it is over. Did you make a basic emotional connection? Were you rushed, blown off or listened to? What was the provider's response to a particular issue or health condition you may have? This is also a very good time to learn how the doctor feels about any non-traditional beliefs you might have. Finally, if you ask a challenging question, watch the manner of the response as much as what is said. This will give important clues as to how future questions will be handled.

Today's health care environment is very stressful for doctors. Finding one who is able to get past the bureaucracy and keep his or her eye on the patient can be difficult. Fortunately, pediatricians manage to do this better than most others. If you find a person who is competent, listens well and puts your child first, realize your good fortune.

c. There are premies and then there are premies

If you know the word exponential, then you might be a math geek like me. If not, you are probably thinking, "Oh no, I bought a math geek's book!" Wait, though, because occasionally math actually does help in the real world. One of those times is with premature babies.

Exponential growth means that a small change in one thing causes a much larger change in another. For example, if you jump off of a ledge, a small change in your time in the air will have a big effect on your speed (thanks to gravity). Jump for one second and you will be fine. Jump for ten seconds- not so much. For a baby, it works the same in reverse: small increases in his time in the womb greatly reduce his risk.

Let's talk numbers. Doctors consider pregnancy to be 40 weeks long (rather than nine months). Babies born *too early* will not make it, but thanks to continuing medical advances, the definition of *too early* keeps being pushed back. Currently, a small percentage of babies as early as 22 weeks gestation can now survive. By 28 weeks, over 90 percent of babies will survive with modern intensive care. A large range of early complications can await these tiny babies. One recent study detected the following, in decreasing order: breathing problems, heart issues, infection, bleeding into the brain, and bowel inflammation (2). Long-term issues can include difficulties in movement known as cerebral pals, as well as learning issues, and vision problems (3).

Between 28 and 32 weeks gestation, the chance of survival starts to inch closer to that of older babies. Non-fatal short and long term complications continue to cause problems, although less with each passing week of maturity. As we discuss elsewhere, there are advantages to getting within a week of the baby's due date, to prevent subtle but important issues.

At this point, you might pause to ask, "How the heck does this chapter make me *Giggle More, Worry Less* ?" That's a very reasonable question. Although discussing this subject provokes anxiety, it is certainly much better to be forewarned, so that you might take steps to avoid premature delivery. The latter would be infinitely more stressful. I guess you could say that avoiding premature delivery will exponentially reduce your stress.

So, how can you avoid premature delivery and all of its issues? In 2014, doctors still do not know the exact reason that labor begins. As, a result, we are forced to do second best, which is to identify and modify factors that put a woman at risk for preterm delivery. These factors include previous preterm delivery, premature contractions, twins and triplets, maternal age and race, obesity, maternal health problems, infections, smoking and other drug use. You will notice that some of these issues can be changed easier than others, and a few not at all.

You have to play the cards that you are dealt. Ideally, everyone can avoid cigarettes and other drugs, and keep a healthy weight. Once you are pregnant, you cannot change your age, race or previous birth history. If you are at high risk, your provider may suggest that you work less or finish earlier, and avoid certain activities. If you develop (or are at risk for) premature labor, doctors may recommend medication to try to stop contractions. Hormonal treatment with progesterone and putting a stitch in the cervix (called *cerclage*) may be recommended. And then there is good old bed rest.

Bed rest was recommended for years as a way to try to postpone delivery. Sandee went through 36 weeks of it, no easy feat for a person who is usually very active. Despite previous widespread use, bed rest to prevent preterm delivery is much less common because there is very little evidence that it works. It does remain an excellent example of the lengths to which parents will go when trying to protect their baby. Most parents would stand on their heads for weeks if their doctor said so. Whatever your doctors might recommend to help your pregnancy, go *all in*. Then you can feel your baby has had the best start that the circumstances allow.

These treatments to prevent preterm delivery can begin at different stages of a pregnancy, depending on your situation. If you have to start before 22 to 24 weeks, you are truly fighting for your baby's survival. After this, each day gives a little better chance for good health. Early on, days matter. Two days of extra maturity will actually impact the baby's outcome. This is one race where the start is more important than the finish. Being extra compliant until 32 weeks is more important than sort of compliant all the way through. The nature of time is that at 28 weeks you can count your gains by half weeks, and at 32, by whole weeks.

Friends and family can have a huge impact on a high-risk mother and vice versa. This is one situation where fathers really can do the work. Most dads will say they can handle holding down the fort much easier than they could handle the baby being delivered too soon. This might help a mother to take it easy, even if she feels like a burden. Older siblings will spend a lot of time with dads and other relatives. They may not understand, but they will be thankful later for a healthy sibling. I admit to a few white lies about how our older kids were doing when we went out. They may have missed Mom, but to hear me talk, they were happy as larks while we were gone.

Sometimes the baby arrives early despite your best efforts. There are a few different ways this can happen. Preterm labor may progress to a point where it cannot be stopped. In these situations, the mother will usually be given a steroid injection, which can help to mature the baby's lungs and reduce newborn complications. Occasionally, a mother's health will not permit her to safely become pregnant; for example, if she has excessively high blood pressure. In this case, the doctor will recommend early delivery as a last resort. What you want to avoid, if possible, is a very early birth away from a hospital that specializes in newborns. Transporting a mother to a specialty hospital before birth is safer than transporting the baby after birth, as long as the mother can safely make it there. Premature birth in an ambulance is not a good plan!

When you eventually get to the newborn intensive care unit (NICU), expect to be overwhelmed. The first sight of tiny babies with so many tubes coming out from them is vivid and scary, even if you have a tour before birth. There is no good way to see your baby like this. You will have to trust and love these highly trained and competent professionals. The viral on-line video journey of Ward Miles explains it better than words (6).

A recent editorial in the journal Pediatrics laments that advances in *treating* premature babies "have not been matched by successes in the efforts to prevent preterm labor and to ensure that pregnancies at risk are carried to satisfactory full-term conclusions."(7) This is a sad truth which hopefully will change soon. Fortunately, victory does not have to be complete to be impactful. Postponing delivery by a few weeks or even days can make a lifetime of difference to a baby. Everyone can appreciate that- math geek or not.

d.   Travel at sic months of pregnancy (and other practical points)

I am lucky enough to live in Cape Cod, MA, a favorite summer vacation destination for many. Pregnant women are among the throngs that descend upon our beaches every year. Unfortunately, some of them go into labor while visiting, much sooner than they expected. We have a very nice community hospital, with good staff and pediatricians. As we discussed, it is not the best place you want to be having a baby 15 weeks early.

Most people avoid travelling close to their due date. This makes sense for social reasons; nesting and such. Having said that, delivery around your due date is incredibly less risky than delivering prematurely. Not that it would be part of your birth plan, but women have done it in rice fields and taxi cabs. So, if you want to have a little getaway before Junior arrives, think about doing it later rather than sooner. Worst-case scenario, you go into labor at the local hospital, which can then handle it just fine. Obviously, isolating yourself is not a winning strategy, so the remote island or campground should wait for another time, as should air travel.

On the subject of travel, mothers are probably the single most safety-conscious group that exists; except, that is, when they are pregnant. Specifically, while pregnant moms wear their seat belts significantly less than the national average (1). Motor vehicle crashes are a leading cause of death for both pregnant women and their fetuses. The American College of Obstetricians and Gynecologists supports seat belt use for pregnant mothers. Just remember, while almost everything is uncomfortable late in pregnancy, lap and shoulder seat belts provide the best protection for mothers and their babies.

Unfortunately, many mothers are in a bit too much of a hurry for the baby to be born. In the past, doctors have been pushed by mothers to schedule an early induction of labor. This is a bad idea. Full gestation for a newborn is 40 weeks. There is now good evidence to suggest that babies born between 34 and 37 weeks gestation (so-called late preterm babies) are four times more likely to have a medical problem and four times as likely to die as term babies. The March of Dimes now encourages all healthy pregnancies to get to at least 39 weeks. Even labors that are induced by the doctor are twice as likely to end up in a C-section. As a close observer, I can tell you that enduring a long labor (sometimes greater than 48 hours) and then having a C-section is like running 25 miles of a marathon, Instead of being allowed to cross the finish line, you are brought for abdominal surgery.

Induction of labor should only be done for good medical reasons, such as high blood pressure, and not for convenience.

OK, so I admit that these are pet peeves, if it wasn't already obvious. Still, they are all-important and will help you and your baby. Thanks for listening!

e. Drugs are bad.

Our society faces many issues, but if I were granted one wish, it would be to get rid of drug and alcohol abuse. As the teacher on the South Park cartoon tells his class, "Drugs are bad."

Pregnancy poses special problems for drug abusers, especially with the drugs known as narcotics or opiates. This includes heroin, but also morphine and oxycodone, for which abuse rates have soared in recent years. Abuse of these drugs usually begins prior to pregnancy, and can be related to dependence developed either from the illegal purchase of these substances, or from prescriptions obtained to treat painful conditions.

Pregnancy is a very bad time to wean off of opiate drugs. Withdrawal during pregnancy leads to an increased risk of death of the fetus. As a result, many pregnant women who seek help with the right intentions are shocked to find out that the best they can do is to have a doctor *manage* their opiate use during the pregnancy.

Increases in opiate use, and problems with stopping opiates during pregnancy have resulted in a boom in births of babies born addicted. In fact, between 2000 and 2010, the number of addicted babies n the United States has tripled. Yes, tripled (1). Not all infants of addicted mothers will develop symptoms, and symptoms are not always determined by how much the mother is using. However, the poor little babies that do develop withdrawal have many of the same symptoms as adults- tremors, sneezing, diarrhea and poor feeding. Most of all they are irritable- inconsolably irritable at times. Untreated, the babies can develop seizures or even die.

Maternity staff can recognize withdrawal symptoms, and scoring systems attempt to assess the symptoms objectively. Some babies will have to be treated with medication, usually a small dose of morphine or some other narcotic. Once the baby improves, the dose is slowly weaned. This process can take a few weeks.

Mothers of addicted babies have to deal with a tremendous amount of guilt. This is understandable, but it can also interfere with the recovery of both the baby and the mother. Mothers have to learn to move forward productively. Cooperation with the resources of the system is important, but it can be difficult, especially if people pass judgment.

All this reinforces the importance of staying drug free in the first place. Drug abuse needs to be dealt with before pregnancy occurs. So often, of course, the opposite is true. Unplanned pregnancy is one of the many consequences of abuse. When pregnancy occurs in an addicted mother, it is especially important for her to get early treatment. This includes not just medication management, but care of the other conditions that often accompany drug use, such as hepatitis and human immunodeficiency virus (HIV).

Narcotics are not the only harmful substance a mother can ingest, although they cause the most obvious withdrawal symptoms. Almost all drugs cross from the mothers system into the fetus. Nicotine and alcohol can reduce a fetus's growth. Alcohol can impair development. The effects on a baby's growth and development depend on the specific drug(s) ingested by the mother. The details of these effects are complicated and fill entire books of their own. Significant issues are known for almost all drugs of abuse.

Like I said, drugs are bad.

Chapter 3: Ready, steady, go

a. Stare at your newborn baby

You have arrived. Planned or unplanned, uneventful or stressful, regular delivery or C-section- Whatever road you took, you have reached your destination. And soon enough, you will be back at home, starting new routines and becoming busy again.

For now, you have two days (or four, if you had a C-section), to recover and to get to know each other. Some of your time will be spent with tasks, especially learning how to feed. Trying to get rest is important, too. This is hard in a hospital, and on a hospital bed, especially if the baby has her days and nights mixed up. Even so, there will be moments when it is quiet and you are undisturbed. This is the ideal opportunity to stare at her.

When you sit back and watch her, you will probably have the incredible realization, "Wow. I made that." Hopefully, you have a partner with whom to share this wonder. If not, your nurse will almost surely be a kindred spirit. The idea of a baby growing inside her mother still seems like a miracle to me. I am still struck that technology cannot replicate the womb as an incubator. Most pregnant mothers can go about their lives: work, do aerobics, have sex and go four-wheel driving, and all the while, that fragile little human being is well-protected.

The next miracle for healthy babies is their ease of adjustment from the womb to the world outside. Within a short time after birth, and a little help in the way of warmth and nutrition, they become comfortable lying in our arms, or laying in a bassinet. Much of this time will be spent sleeping, but there will be periods when a newborn lays quietly awake and calm.

This *quiet awake* stage is a great time to watch your baby. If the room is sufficiently warm, she can be unswaddled, and partially undressed. Check out her fingers and toes- see whose they resemble. Some have skinny *chicken* legs, and others are stocky. You can see her move in the basinet. Her legs will likely be bent from months of living in tight quarters. Her arms will probably be on either side of her head. Hands may open, then close again. Her movements may seem disorganized- she is testing out how her parts work.

Some will have full thick heads of hair, and others hardly any. There is nothing softer than newborn hair. Look at her face. Most Caucasian babies have blue eyes at first. Darker skinned babies will have darker eyes. Newborns can see about two feet in front of them – just the right distance from a mother while feeding. Amazingly, when studied by researchers, a two-day-old baby would rather stare at her mother's face than any other person (1).

Sometimes babies will yawn, sneeze or hiccough. One of my old professors used to say that a yawning baby is a happy baby.

Newborns have funny breathing patterns. Their normal breathing rate is about 40 to 60 times per minute, more than twice that of an adult. Most of the time it is regular and rhythmic, but not always. *Periodic breathing* is a normal pattern where the breathing alternates from shallow and panting to actual pauses of up to about five seconds. This can freak you out as a parent if you are not expecting it. The key is that the baby remains nice and pink, oblivious to our concerns.

How you choose to capture these moments is up to you. Personally, I am a fan of mental snapshots, but certainly many people love video. I would encourage you to limit your visitors and your electronic contact to those who are truly important. Remember, the more people who are around, the less one-on-one time you get with your baby.

This is a rare and special moment in your life. It can be one you remember forever if you take the time to savor it.

b. How to succeed in breastfeeding without it being trying.

It is a little stressful, as a man, to write a chapter on breastfeeding. The finer points of nursing mechanics are left to the experts; that is, the lactation consultants. Having said that, 20 years of observation of the process of nursing leaves me with some thoughts that you might find valuable.

My approach is undoubtedly shaped by my wife's experience nursing our three children, especially Catherine, our oldest. At that point, I had lots of theoretical knowledge and no practical experience. We lived far from our families. Our friends had been very helpful during a difficult pregnancy, and we did not want to trouble them for more help. Sandee came home on day 3 with our beautiful, mildly jaundiced baby girl. As usual, her milk had yet to come in. When the milk arrived, it did so with a bang, Sandee became engorged and Catherine was unable to feed effectively. I went out to get a breast pump, having no clue what one looked like. What a nightmare! Somehow, my two girls worked through these struggles, and a long and successful period of nursing followed.

How much easier it was the next two times! Sandee had experience, and more importantly, confidence in how to nurse. We had also moved to Falmouth, and gained access to Linda Sayers, a local lactation consultant par excellence, who was more than happy to help Sandee. From then on, I bowed down to Linda for helping us. Since that time, she and her partners have given great advice to thousands of mothers in our area.

I hope that the importance of breast milk and breastfeeding is now common knowledge. Breastfeeding is complete nutrition for a newborn (with the exception of Vitamin D and sometimes additional iron, which the doctor may recommend). Breast fed babies are less likely to develop recurrent ear infections, pneumonia, diarrheal illnesses, asthma, eczema, obesity and diabetes. They are less likely to die of Sudden Infant Death Syndrome (SIDS). For mothers, it lowers the future rates of breast and ovarian cancer, and promotes healthy weight loss, in addition to promoting mother-child bonding (1).

If parents schedule a pediatrician prenatal visit, we ask about feeding. These first-time parents often say that they are "going to try to" breastfeed. This comment speaks volumes. It expresses both their desire to nurse, and their anxiety about succeeding. Health care providers need to promote breastfeeding. We need to have adequate lactation supports in place to help new mothers, and we need to be honest about the process. Breastfeeding is not a point and click phenomenon. It is a tried-and-true old-fashioned pump, which takes a few days to prime. We do women a disservice by giving the impression that the baby will spring from the womb, leap to the breast and everyone will live happily ever after. This sets up mothers for feelings of failure and low self esteem; never a good thing, but especially not in the first week post partum.

Women who plan to breastfeed should be aware of one controversial issue regarding their pain control in labor and its effect on breastfeeding. Again, this is a perilous area for a man to address. Essentially, it has been *proposed* that medication that the mother receives in her epidural can get across to the baby and interfere with the baby's ability to begin breastfeeding. Studies in this area are difficult to perform, because many factors contribute to breastfeeding success, and it is hard to single out just one. Not surprisingly, this has lead to conflicting results. Some advocates feel that even raising the subject can create guilt surrounding a woman's right to adequate pain control, and ignores the impact of pain on a mother's psyche. In 2014, the issue has not been resolved. Perhaps this allows an individual mother the freedom to determine how much medicine is right for her, as she and her infant embark on labor together. She can pick the pain control that will put her and her baby in a place to have a successful first feeding soon after birth.

After the important initial feeding, mothers and their babies continue on a feeding adventure lasting several days. Most of the work is up the baby. The ideal situation is a healthy, hungry baby who is alert but calm, and who has a strong suck reflex. A mother can facilitate feeding by staying calm and determined. Problems can almost always be overcome with help, as long as you stick with it.

Nursing takes time. The main goal is to have the pump up and running well by the end of a week. Although a few babies get it right away, the much more typical pattern can be broken down by day. On day 1, after the birth experience, the baby is tired and the mother is tired. On day 2, the baby gets hungry, often very hungry and wants to feed a lot, sometimes almost continuously. This cluster feeding can be exhausting. Many times the baby will be fussy; parents often misinterpret this as *gassy*, when it is really just hunger. The second night is often long. By day 3, the milk comes in for fortunate mothers; for most others, it comes in day 4. The first time that your baby has that *drunk on milk* look is a great moment- you know he has what he needs and you can breathe a sigh of relief.

As we discussed, preterm babies are often slow feeders. They are often sleepy and can be hard to wake up to feed well. This can happen with term babies, too. The cycle of sleepiness and slow feeding can build upon itself, since inadequate nutrition leads to low strength, more sleeping, poor feeding and so on. These babies have to be pushed with sponge baths, wet washcloths, and other reasonable ways of try to rouse the baby (a thorough exam by the pediatrician never hurts either, both to make sure all is well, and to rouse a sleepy baby- they are almost all crying by the time I finish with them!)

During these early days, most parents these days obsess about numbers: their babies weight (essentially all babies lose weight the first couple or few days), and what percentage he has lost, as well as the number of poops and pees. To me, this is more often counterproductive than it is productive. To begin with, babies having been living in water for the previous nine months; they come out a little waterlogged and for this reason, losing some weight in the first couple of days is part of the normal process. This stops by about the third day, and it is true that excessive weight loss after this time can be a sign of concern. However, this is for the nurses and doctors to worry about, not the parents. The mother's job is to feed and care for her baby. When parents get too caught up in the numbers, it can have the same effect as watching the stock market too closely- a small decline can lead to panic.

Fathers have an important role to play and *not* to play during the initiation of nursing. We provide moral support, give our partners a good person to hand the baby to so she can rest, whether it is for diaper changes, burping or just to hold and bounce. We are also the gophers. Most of us try to be helpful. When we get too involved in the actual nursing, we start to run the risk of interfering. One pediatrician/friend used to say that nursing is as close to feelings about a woman's womanhood as impotence is to a man's manhood. You can imagine how a guy would feel in the latter situation if a woman kept helpfully asking, "How's it going?"

Sometimes it is necessary to supplement the baby's feeding, preferably with pumped breast milk. To be honest, most parents, and many physicians and nurses are too quick to supplement. This can happen when any of us make decisions too much on the numbers-weight loss, pees and poops- rather than by listening to the baby (one exception to this is a low blood sugar, which is not something to mess around with; it needs immediate attention to avoid problems for the baby.) There is no one right time to say when a supplement is needed. It depends on the full assessment of the baby and the mother's milk, and is best left to the good judgment of the healthcare team in consultation with the parents. This is one time that providers need to give clear guidance to the parents about the right decision. Every mother will be worried about her baby's hunger. She will not feel comfortable waiting to supplement without clear reassurance from the doctor or nurse.

There is no shortage of unsolicited advice about feeding. Breastfeeding is a classic *too many cooks* problem. I highly recommend finding one provider who becomes your breastfeeding advisor, and sticking with her. If you have access to a lactation consultant, it is ideal to meet her while you are still in the hospital. If this isn't possible, or if you don't work together well, there will likely be a maternity nurse whose advice seems to be the most helpful. In this case, find out when she is working in the week after discharge. That way, if you need to call, you can pick up where you left off the last time. Having to start from scratch with a new person can be very frustrating and counterproductive. Remember, you don't need to know every breastfeeding position, just one that works, and a second as backup.

At hospital discharge, my parting words to new nursing mothers usually include, "Remember, billions have gone before you." It is a system that has stood the test of time. However, to ensure success, a mother will need continued support. This is a big issue in North America, but we are making progress, thanks largely to an increase in lactation consultants. Initial breastfeeding rates are up to 79 percent, and six-month rates to 49 percent. With a good team around you, the challenges of breastfeeding can definitely be overcome. Go in positive and stay strong. Once you achieve success, it can become one of the most rewarding parts of motherhood for this baby and his future siblings.

c.   Holding your baby grows his brain, it does not spoil him

My mother says that if I hold my baby too much I will spoil him. Is this true?

This is still one of the most common questions at the first or second visit to the pediatrician. You know it is a real source of conflict when the grandmother shows up with the mother.

Short answer: No, it is good for a baby to be held. It promotes social brain growth.

Long answer: Many parents from previous generations were taught that holding a baby too much would teach the baby to expect to be held, and somehow spoil them. This notion dates back to at least Victorian times, according to Dr. Spock, author of *the* parenting book, <u>The Common Sense Book of Baby and Child Care</u>, which for 50 years, was so influential that only the Bible sold more copies. Spock explains that several factors, from advances in educational and developmental psychology, to Freudian fears about sexuality (when children feel abandoned by their mothers) led to a gradual understanding that it is good to hold a child. Most of all, lack of parental attention was shown to have adverse outcomes in later life.

Of course, the natural instincts of parents tell us to hold our babies. What new mother wants to sit and listen to her baby cry? As my neighbor used to say, "Crying is a perfectly designed sound. It gets immediate attention". It turns out that, as usual, Mother Nature was right. Holding a baby helps to grow a baby's brain. Premature babies that are held *kangaroo* style have better weight gain, less infections, and other complications than those that are looked after in other ways. Babies who are held more early on also appear to be better adjusted once they reach the toddler years.

From a parent's perspective, holding your baby is important for your piece of mind, but for other reasons, too. I have watched many parents over the years stand by while I examined their newborn. Almost inevitably, the baby is crying by the time I finish. New parents have an understandably hard with this. At times, the crying can be for a few minutes, as when I need to draw blood. This is like torture- crying is distressing on a very physical and emotional level.

I try very hard not to have any discussion with a parent while her baby is crying. It is just about impossible to listen to anything other than the baby. Go figure. (Yes, I am a pediatrician and had to learn this the hard way!) At home, it can be equally difficult to not respond to what you think your baby needs.

We know that a baby's crying affects how parents cope. Colicky babies are at more risk for child abuse, and their mothers are at higher risk for depression. For most parents, the baby's crying is not the main factor involved, but it sure doesn't help. On a lesser scale, even happy families will be happier when the baby cries less.

In the past, some people were very intent on getting the baby on a *schedule*, in other words, set times to eat and sleep. These days, we usually let the baby call the shots, since a baby knows best, and everyone is happier. There are a few exceptions- some newborns are sleepy and have to be prodded to wake up and eat. Twins and other *multiples* usually need to be fed around the same time just for their parents' sanity. Sometimes, a parent's personality is such that schedules are necessary. If you are super organized and need a little more control, there is nothing wrong with this. The take-home message is that you do not need to let your new baby cry if you want to hold her.

By holding your baby when he needs or wants it, you are teaching him that he is important. He learns she is loved and can trust that her basic needs will be met. As a parent, it helps you to feel good.

It also allows you to be guilt-free when you need to let her cry- like when you are in the bathroom, busy with something else, or when you just need five minutes to sit.

And what about spoiling? Believe me, I do not advocate spoiling a child. The key is to understand what spoils them. Love, attention and affection are good for a child. Children become spoiled when they are older and their parents are unable or unwilling to consistently say "No" to some of the child's requests. As I like to say, in the first year you learn you are the center of the universe, and in years two through eighteen, you learn there are a few other stars out there, too- including your mom and dad.

d. Mothers: listen to your babies; fathers listen to the mothers

OK, I know people are going to give me a lot of grief for this one, but what the heck.

After 25 years of experience, it continues to impress me that, when it comes to spousal disputes about the baby, mothers are almost always right. I'm sorry, guys; the truth hurts. I throw myself into this group, too, with the possible exception of issues of medical knowledge. I have no idea how much of this is genetic and how much is learned, but mothers just seem to get it right much more often than we do.

The extent to which some new mothers know every detail of her baby's appearance can be astounding, and I think the same is true for his voice, breathing, facial expressions and so on. While part of this comes from proximity, I can't help but think there is a connection on a deeper level. I suspect that this is connected to why mothers can tell when something is wrong with the baby. It is as if the baby is an actual extension of the mother.

Fathers and babies, on the other hand, do not generally have this same kind of cosmic bond. Most of us are downright afraid of hurting the baby at first, which is natural, but surprisingly unfounded. Some are disinterested and others are absent. Most of us have little to no experience with newborns. Even the best of fathers usually pales next to his wife/partner when it comes to nurturing skills. And that is OK, too, as long as we are trying our best.

Having said that, many of us guys are surprisingly willing to offer opinions that have no basis in knowledge, experience or intuition, just because, well, we think it. It is sometimes impressive how confident guys can be, when we are absolutely wrong. Perhaps natural selection has found confidence to be a generally useful adaptive mechanism. I don't know.

As a general rule, mothers should listen to their babies and fathers should listen to the mothers. I do not mean this as any kind of put-down to men; it is just that, in our society, this is what works. Of course, dads should listen to the babies, too and share our thoughts with our wives/girlfriends. Mothers should not be condescending to us and make us feel that we are not valued or useful. However, if in doubt, a tie vote goes to the mother. And fathers with natural confidence can use that confidence to support mothers who have the knowledge but doubt themselves.

There will be exceptions. For some couples, the father will truly be the more observant one. Occasionally, a mother's emotional condition prevents her from being objective. Sometimes the father will have had experience as an older brother of many siblings, or having had children in a previous relationship. He might have medical or other training that gives us opinions based on knowledge. Sometimes, on special days, the rest of us schmucks will just plain old get it right.

And when that happens, as one dad put it, we should *self celebrate.*

e.   Fourth day crying- a perfectly incongruent storm

"It's sunny outside!"
 "My husband made me pancakes!"
Both of these proclamations were made by mothers who were crying their eyes out at well check-ups. Both said they that what were feeling underneath was, "I'm so happy. Why am I crying?" If

you have or had a similar experience, it's okay. You are not going crazy. This is a phenomenon I call *fourth day crying*.

While <u>The Perfect Storm</u>, by Sebastian Junger, originally described an event that happened at sea, the journey that you take as a new parent is full of emotional crests and troughs. These collide on or about the fourth day after birth. To begin, a woman's body is in the midst of a huge hormonal shift. Think about having someone living inside of you, and then no longer living there. What kind of a transition must be occurring in your body? Add to this the feelings of worry and responsibility that come with parenthood, and the fatigue which is undoubtedly growing. Put them all together and you have the all the necessary ingredients for a storm. And this is being optimistic.

There are so many other factors that can pile on top. This is the time when breast milk is usually *coming in*, which has its own set of worries and hormones. It is also when newborn jaundice may be a worry. There are many other issues which could have developed for a mother or baby, and I haven't even mentioned any of the emotional stressors which a new baby seems to aggravate. All in all, some crying is completely appropriate.

And yet, none of these factors address the true mystery of this condition. What sets fourth day crying apart is that the tears usually come on without warning, when you are happy. I would even speculate one step further. As an observer, it is not a regular happiness, not laughing to the point of tears. It gives the appearance of a strangely euphoric happiness. This is why I call the emotions incongruent. They don't seem like they should fit together, except that so many women experience it.

Fourth day crying is a little different than *post partum blues*, with which most people are familiar. Post partum blues tends to happen over a broader span of time and it is associated with being sad. We use this term for the common sadness that many mothers feel, and which can progress to true depression.

Once you understand fourth day crying, you can breathe a sigh of relief. You are not going crazy. Your partner will probably be relieved, too. There is also humor in it. In my estimation, any humor injected into this otherwise stressful time is a very good thing.

And I wish I could make the pancakes good enough to bring you tears.

f.   Don't try to prevent grandparents from spoiling your child

Becoming a grandparent is the reward that you get for all of the work you do as a parent.

Think about everything that you are going through in your first year of parenthood. Now multiply that by your age, and you will get a sense of what grandparents are bringing to this point in their lives. This is a truly special time for them, and one that is usually well earned.

I have yet to witness post-grandmother depression. Every grandmother I have ever met is absolutely thrilled by the arrival of a new baby. That is not to say that all of them are happy to hear about their daughter's pregnancy, especially when it is unplanned. However, when the time comes for the baby to arrive, any ill feelings seem to be long forgotten. I hope that all mothers can share the joy of a new baby with an involved grandmother, because this is a special gift.

There will, of course, be times when mothers and grandmothers differ in their opinions about what is best for the baby. Many child-rearing practices have changed, and sometimes the differences between old and new recommendations can be a source of conflict. I am always amazed by how well grandmothers remember what *Dr. Smith* told them thirty years ago. Sometimes I hope my advice is not taken that much to heart! In any case, a good grandmother will defer to her daughter most of the time. If there is an issue, the pediatrician can be the bad cop, so that you can say *the doctor said…*.

When you have a new baby and are living with your mother, this can be a blessing or a curse, or sometimes both. You will know into which group you fit. Good grandmothers are a gift to the entire family. However, difficult grandmothers can make it hard for you to be a mother and a daughter in the same house. These grandmothers will insist on doing it *their* way. Any attempts to dissuade them are likely to be met with, "Well, you turned out OK, didn't you?"

Conflicts with grandparents are never more present than when it comes to spoiling. I think it is very difficult for those of us who are not grandparents to imagine the bond that they feel towards their grandchildren. It seems as if they are pulled like a large magnet, which they have neither the strength nor the desire to resist. Part of this pull is to please, and spoiling is the means to this end.

I try to think of this from the child's perspective. When my daughter, Catherine, was five, she returned from a visit to her grandparents' house with a *secret*. We asked, "Do we know the secret?"

"Nope", she replied.

"Does Grandma know the secret?"

"Yes ", she smiled. "Only the people that give me Diet Coke know the secret." All of us should be so lucky as to have someone that spoils us (as long as it is not our parents.) Kids are certainly smart enough to know that they can get away with things with their grandparents. Again, that does become problematic when the grandmother is living with you or doing a large share of the daytime caregiving. These are very important conflicts to resolve, mostly for the sake of your sanity. Unfortunately, the grandparents who are least in sync with your parenting wishes are likely to be the hardest ones to convince to alter their behavior. Your circumstances, that is, your reliance on them for housing and childcare, may dictate that you are the one who does the bending. This is really difficult to do, but may be the only option, except for moving out.

Grandfathers are not as consistent in their behavior as grandmothers. We all know the stereotypes, from the grumpy old man that you do not want to bother, to the kind, playful soul whose lap the kids compete to sit on. Many new grandfathers are in their forties and fifties, and do not fit this mold at all. I see a lot of older men who play essential roles in the family's day-to-day life. It is not unusual for a man to be considerably more mellow and involved as a grandfather than he was as a father. I'm not sure if is increased maturity, decreased testosterone, more free time or all of the above.

All too commonly of late, grandparents are assuming the primary parenting role. This is most often due to parental substance abuse, although there are many other reasons. These grandparents have my undying respect. I try to imagine how challenging it must be to be performing all of a parent's duties when you should be enjoying *yourself*. Most do it out of love, and because they cannot stand the thought of their grandchild going into foster care. I have seen more than one grandparent ultimately have to refuse the care of a third or fourth grandchild, because an unfit mother continues to have children. This must be truly agonizing.

My children have been blessed with four fantastic grandparents, who have all stayed healthy until at least their late seventies. Through getting to know, enjoying, learning from and being spoiled by my parents and in-laws, they have received a perspective on life that just would not be possible without them. These perspectives will stay with them forever. I hope that you can have this good fortune, and can turn a blind eye when Grandpa sneaks them a little extra ice cream.

g.   To be or not to be....circumcised: that is the question

Circumcision is a very personal subject, and a very personal decision. It takes into account medical, cultural, religious and social values. For some people, it is an easy decision. For most of us, it requires a careful consideration of pros and cons.

In the present day, the main medical issues are straightforward. Circumcised boys have a lower rate of urinary tract infection, but this is still relatively uncommon. Circumcised men in Africa have a lower rate of developing HIV, but condoms also have this effect. There is a lower rate of penile cancer in circumcised men, but this is rare, and we don't go cutting off other parts of the body to prevent cancer unless the risk is exceedingly high. Finally, nurses will tell horror stories about the difficulties that old uncircumcised men can have in the nursing home. Again, you could argue about the logic of a preemptive operation to prevent a possible outcome seventy- plus years later. The down side is subjecting anyone, let alone a newborn to *unnecessary* surgery, which always carries a small risk of infection or bleeding.

Pain control should not be a factor. With local anesthetics and sugar to suck on, most boys should be comfortable during the procedure. I have been doing circumcisions my entire practice life and can honestly say that the majority get through it really well. I'm sure the occasional one has a local that doesn't work well. Some scream because they don't like being held down, or for reasons unrelated to the procedure. Some fall asleep. I often encourage a family member to be present if they are up to it, so they can see that it is much easier on their boy than most imagine (this is by no means mandatory- the last thing you want is a father passing out while you are in mid-circumcision! I also usually discourage mothers from attending, feeling that they have done enough work in the previous 48 hours, but that's just me.)

The social part of the decision is, well, less cut and dry. Is it important for a boy's penis to resemble his father's penis? Or his brother's? Some people would say yes; others would say that family members have different color hair and nobody thinks twice about it. Is it important to look like the other boys in the locker room

72

during high school? There is always something about each of us that is different from the crowd, but on the other hand, high school can be difficult enough without getting teased about your penis. I have had a few boys come to me as teenagers requesting circumcision purely for social reasons, and there is no question that if you are going to circumcise, the newborn period is easier than adolescence or adulthood.

A lot people in North America misunderstand care of the uncircumcised penis. Essentially, prior to the foreskin becoming retractile, there is *no* care required. Many times parents will question the development of white material at the tip of the foreskin or under it. This is called *smegma-* it is a natural lubricant and is normal. Sometimes it can clump up, which I refer to as a *smegma ball* - it is equally harmless.

The foreskin becomes retractile at its own pace, which can be well past age ten. If it is not causing any problem for the boy, then there is nothing to do at that time. Once it is retractile, gentle retraction, cleansing and then bringing the skin back down helps to prevent infection and is recommended. That's really it.

One unfortunate trend in circumcised boys is their parents' obsession with making sure that no part of the foreskin is attached to or covering any part of the head of the penis. This is really not of any importance and a redo circumcision to correct this is not necessary. The same thing goes for any sloppiness of the circumcision skin edge. Mothers and fathers tend to worry about this on theoretical *less than perfect* basis, but I can assure you that nobody is really going to care about it later. Any pediatrician will tell you that there is no one typical appearance, just like any other part of the body.

Finally, there is a subject that is very difficult to discuss with an individual parent, but which is good to know about. Once in a while, I drag my feet about doing a circumcision because the penis is small. This is probably in part because circumcising a small penis is more technically difficult. Mostly though, it is the concept of *Do No Harm* that is part of a doctor's oath. I have no idea if there is a correlation between penis size at birth and in adulthood. I do know that sometimes it is really hard to do a proper circumcision without removing most of the skin of the penis, especially on the underside near the scrotum. And somehow, that doesn't seem right. However, it is a bigger wrong for me to make a parent feel bad by saying, "You know, I think your son's penis is too small to circumcise". This would scar the parent for life and probably it would affect the boy somehow.

Whichever decision you make, try not to dwell. After all, it is like a haircut- you can't decide to put it back after it has been cut.

h. A happy baby for a week is a happy baby for a week.

On the other hand, a happy baby for three weeks is a happy baby.

These were the words of the God of Child Development, Dr. T. Berry Brazelton. He is making a few points with this statement. First of all, many babies are relatively content in the first few days. Most babies are tired after labor and delivery just like their mothers. They can sleep twenty hours or more out of twenty-four. Most of their awake time is spent feeding, which is usually a happy time once they start to get enough to eat. And there is usually a competition to hold the newborn, which is something that most babies like. Still, most newborns are primarily just mellow compared to the rest of us.

Some stay that way and some do not. If you think about it, in a week a baby becomes seven times older than he was at birth. For adults to live to seven times our current age would be several lifetimes. Thought of this way, it is no wonder that a lot of changes occur. More practically, the situations that tend to make babies unhappy commonly begin in the second week. The first of these is that a one week old is already considerably more alert than he was at birth. The more time you are awake, the more time you have to be unhappy. If he is allergic to or not tolerant of his milk, these symptoms take at least a few days to develop. A baby with excessive spitting or gastro-esophageal reflux will start to develop more throat irritation by this time. Bottle fed babies have had time to become constipated, if they are prone. Breast fed babies, which are almost never constipated, can still have the normal cramping before passing stool, which can also lead to crying.

Factors at home can lead to more crying too. Parents are usually exhausted by the end of week one. Family members may be around less to help. This can lead to less time with the baby being held, and more upset. The presence of young siblings or other family members can lead to a more chaos. Sometimes the baby will just be impatient when he has to wait for his feeding or changing. New evidence also suggests that *some* babies who cry a lot are more prone to migraine headaches as older children (1).

And then there is plain old colic, which is what pediatricians call prolonged bouts of crying for which there is no good explanation. We will talk more about this later, but this, too, seems to kick in after the honeymoon period of the first week.

So, if you get through the first week in good shape, it is cause for thanks. If you get three weeks under your belt, you can usually breathe a sigh of relief. Even if you do not, as the Buddhists say, "All conditioned things are impermanent. Strive on with diligence." (2)

i.   Newborn jaundice: my gal or fellow is yellow

Catherine is my first-born. Now twenty, she was four days old and pretty as a picture in her white outfit, as I went off to run some errands. On my return, she had been changed into a yellow sleeper. This brought out the jaundice in her skin. When I was unusually quiet at dinner, Sandee knew something was up. "What's wrong?" she asked.

"She's jaundiced", I reluctantly admitted.

"What does that mean for her?" was the obvious next question.

Sandee may have been the first to ask that question of me, but she certainly was not the last. Most lay people have heard of newborn jaundice, but very few understand it, although they suspect it has something to do with the liver.   Even fewer people realize why pediatricians are so interested in it. To answer these questions, we need a short newborn physiology tutorial.

When a baby is inside her mother, she gets her oxygen from her mother's blood, which comes across the placenta (or afterbirth) and then into the baby's circulation. Oxygen is taken up and delivered to the baby by her red blood cells. This specialized task requires a specialized red blood cell. When the baby is born, she begins to get oxygen through her lungs. The specialized red blood cell is no longer required, and the body gradually gets rid of them. The red blood cell pigment is converted to the yellow pigment known as bilirubin, which has to be eliminated from the body. The body eliminates bilirubin by processing it in the liver and sending it to the stool, where it can be pooped out. This high volume of bilirubin takes a while to be excreted. In the meantime, the body will develop a yellow hue, known as jaundice (fun fact: jaune is the French word for yellow.)

In moderation, newborn jaundice is a normal process. Scientists even believe that some bilirubin helps with baby's transition from to low oxygen inside the mother to higher oxygen after birth, by acting as what is called an antioxidant (1). However, too much bilirubin can lead to problems. Excess jaundice happens when too many blood cells are broken down, or the body is unable to get rid of enough bilirubin. The most serious form of red blood cell breakdown happens when a mother's blood reacts against the baby's blood cells. Think of our blood type as putting badges on the coat of our red blood cells. At one extreme, AB Positive red blood cells will have three badges, one each for A, B and Rh positive. At the other extreme, O Negative blood type cells will have no badges. When a mother is negative for the badge, and the baby is positive, the mother can make what is called an antibody to the baby's cells, which can cross into the baby's circulation, leading to increased and prolonged breakdown. This scenario is most serious when a mother is Rh negative and a baby is Rh positive, which is why Rh negative mothers get a shot called *Rhogam* during the pregnancy. It can also occur with discrepancies in A and B, and even other lesser-known badges. These situations are usually discovered early, because high-risk maternal blood types get tested for a reaction. Occasionally, early, severe jaundice leads to the discovery.

Less severe forms of jaundice happen for a variety of reasons. These include excess bruising leading to increased breakdown of red blood cells, slow onset of breastfeeding, leading to less bowel movements, and prematurity, where everything works a little less efficiently.

Returning to Catherine, she developed mild jaundice at a typical time, about day four. Her jaundice was first noticed in the face and eye whites. As jaundice progresses, it tends to move down the body to the chest and eventually the legs. Most people are not good at recognizing jaundice. Catherine's grandfather insisted that she (and eventually her brothers) were olive-skinned, even though Sandee is a rosy-cheeked Celt and I have lily-white English skin.

Twenty years ago, most of the initial testing was done by the doctor's eyeball. We were fortunate to have Dr. Bob Connolly, a residency friend that didn't mind a knock on his door at 10 pm. It was a brief conversation. "Bob, tell us that Catherine is fine", we half-asked, half-told him.
"She's fine", was the reply.
"Thanks. Good night."
He allowed us to get some much-needed sleep that night.

Most parents do not have this luxury. Fortunately, most hospital nurseries will now test the baby before discharge, either with a blood test, or with a meter that estimates the jaundice level through the skin. Your doctor should let you know at discharge whether your baby is expected to be safe, at routine or higher risk. Remember that the process peaks somewhere around day 4 to 6, which is before a one week old well doctor visit. Often times, an arrangement is made for the baby to be tested after discharge, seen by a visiting nurse, or scheduled for an early doctor visit.

Why do we care about jaundice so much, anyway? Many doctors tend to leave this out of our explanations. The truth is, at very high levels, bilirubin can deposit into the brain, leading to a permanent injury to areas that control movement. This condition, known as kernicterus, is thankfully rare, but it still does occur on occasion. It is always a tragedy. By keeping the jaundice level under a peak of 20 or so (in US units), the chances of this are greatly reduced. In fact, even above this level, most babies are fine; we do not fully understand which ones are at increased risk.

Now that you are petrified, you can relax. While it is true that a little knowledge can be dangerous, it is equally true that a healthy respect for a potential problem is safer than ignorance.

And if you are still worried, remember you share company even with pediatricians who are new parents.

Chapter 4: Intestinal fortitude

a. Spit happens

Sandee bought me a brown leather jacket shortly after we were married. It was really nice and I used to wear it a lot. When Andrew (our middle child) came along, he spit up more in one day than our other two did in their whole first year. Eventually, you-know-who had christened every piece of clothing I owned, including the jacket. I still have it, and you can still see the stain on the left shoulder.

Spitting up is common and usually harmless. Most mothers are very familiar with heartburn, the feeling of your stomach contents coming back into your throat. With babies, it goes a step further and comes out the mouth. Sometimes it even comes out the nose, which freaks people out, even though this is just physics.

A lot of people are unclear about the difference between spitting up and throwing up. I explain it differently than most doctors. To me, most spitting up gives no warning- one minute the baby is fine and the next milk is coming up, just like heartburn for the mother. In contrast, vomiting happens when you are not feeling good. For a baby, this usually involves a period of fussiness before the fluid comes up.

Gastro-esophageal reflux, also known as GERD, is really just exaggerated spitting up. Technically, there isn't a big difference. Practically, it is a matter of degree. If the amount of laundry is the main problem, then I am happy to still call it spitting up. If the spitting causes a complication, then doctors call it reflux. By complication, we think of poor weight gain, choking spells or persistent crying. Persistent crying is caused by irritation to the esophagus (the tube between the throat and the stomach), from acid repeatedly going up and down it. This will cause some babies will be poor sleepers. Others will arch their backs repeatedly.

There are several red flags that should make parents and doctors consider a condition more serious than reflux. The main concerns are green (bile) or red/black (blood) vomit. Projectile vomiting occurs when the fluid comes out forcefully. Spit-up usually lands on your shoulder. Projectile vomiting goes over your shoulder. One father I know compared it to the *The Exorcist* (you can use your imagination if you haven't seen it). The take-home message is that projectile vomiting can indicate a blockage, and should prompt a visit to the doctor. Green or bloody vomiting can be a medical emergency.

Reflux in babies is *not* usually caused by what she is drinking; that is, the breast milk or formula. This is a common misconception, partly because reflux tends to happen after eating, and perhaps because adult reflux is sometimes related to diet. When a baby has a problem with what she eats, other symptoms are usually present, such as fussiness and diarrhea. This means that multiple formula changes are likely to get you nowhere but frustrated when your baby has just reflux.

Sometimes it can be hard to tell the difference between reflux and breast milk/ formula allergy. Not all babies are at one extreme (happy but refluxing) or the other (fussy, gassy, vomiting, with loose, mucusy or bloody stools). Sometimes it is a challenge, even for doctors. We look for clues, the same way a detective tries to build a case against a suspect. If a happy baby has problems mainly when she is laid down, reflux is more suspicious. On the other hand, if a fussy baby has other signs of allergy, especially eczema on the skin, we wonder about allergy. Sometimes we have to test our theory by treating one or the other to get a better answer. Occasionally, in a truly colicky baby, or one who is losing weight, we treat for both. This *shoot first, ask questions later* approach is reserved for severe situations, when we don't have the luxury of a step-wise approach.

Once we diagnose reflux, how do we make it stop? Even if you do nothing, it will usually start to improve about 6 months of age. You may notice temporary steps backwards when she is teething or has a cold. In addition to time, feeding techniques are often useful. Mothers become experts in when their baby needs to stop for a minute, or be burped, or which bottle nipple seems to help the best. This is no surprise when you consider that a baby will be fed over 500 times in the first six months.

The next steps can be thought of in two groups- first, we want to make less milk come up. Next, we want to reduce the acid content of milk that does come up, to reduce irritation. There are two old - fashioned ways of making less food come up- thickening feedings with cereal, and elevating the head of the crib. Both of these make common sense, but unfortunately neither seems to work very well, at least according to medical studies. I must admit to still recommending them, in part because they just seem logical and because there is very little to lose. Formula can be thickened with up to 1 *tablespoon* (not teaspoon) of cereal for every 2 ounces of formula. Rice has traditionally been used, but lately some people are using oatmeal. We watch to make sure this cereal doesn't cause constipation. Sometimes parents have to change to a larger hole in the bottle nipple. Cereal also boosts the calories/ounce of formula and it is important to watch for excess weight gain, too.

Elevating the head of the crib is a little trickier. Mattresses can be raised up with books under the baby's head area or with wedges that can be purchased. Pillows should never be placed on the mattress. To avoid the baby sliding down to the bottom, *Velcro* harnesses can be used. Harnessing the baby avoids her ending up crumpled in a ball down at the lower end of the crib. Any product you use should be approved for safety. There are potential concerns with sliding in between a wedge and the side of a crib.

Refluxing babies should still be placed on their BACKS to sleep. The risk of SIDS is important and the risk of choking spit-up from back sleeping is thankfully very low.

The main treatment for most refluxers is medication, especially those that reduce acid production by the stomach. Adults may be familiar with the names ranitidine (*Zantac*), omeprazole (*Prilosec*) and pantoprazole (*Prevacid*) (1). The medicines are given to babies in liquid form, and do not taste the best. Giving a bad tasting medicine to a spitty baby leads to some challenges. With perseverance (and sometimes flavoring), this can usually be overcome. Most babies do very well on these medicines.

I would say more, but I think its time to get that spit-up stain off of my leather jacket.

b. Got milk problems?

One of the pleasures of writing a book is the chance to thoroughly explain a subject that always seems a little rushed in a well child checkup. Infant feeding is definitely one of those areas.

For starters, let's think about a two-week-old baby who is fussy. He could be either breast or formula fed, and he cries a lot, especially after eating. He occasionally throws up and he is not constipated. His weight gain has been good. You come to see me, and we decide that his diet is the most likely reason for his fussiness.

At this point, doctors think about whether the problem is a true allergy, or more of what we call intolerance. Parents often confuse the two terms, or maybe it is not important what it is called as long as it is fixed! Understanding the difference matters, because it changes how we try to make the baby better.

True allergies in the body are mounted towards proteins. A food allergy is a reaction against a specific protein being consumed. For babies, the most common offender is one of the milk proteins. Regular infant formulas are *milk-based*; that is, the major proteins used are from cow's milk, namely casein and whey. The mix of casein and whey may vary from formula to formula, but these two proteins are the main suspects for causing allergy. A true milk protein allergy requires a switch to a non-dairy formula.

Many babies will be changed to soy formula. Still, about one third of babies with a true milk allergy will also have an allergy to soy protein. These babies will need to drink a *hypoallergenic* formula, which means low allergy. Hypoallergenic formulas usually have broken down the proteins to smaller molecules. Smaller molecules are less prone to stimulate an allergic response.

Breast fed babies, in general, have less difficulty with allergy. This is true not just while nursing, but also throughout childhood, and is yet another reason why breast milk is such a good thing. Breast milk contains more than just calories. It also contains factors which improve the baby's immune system. Occasionally, though, a baby can be allergic to some component of the breast milk. Cow's milk ingested by the mother can make its way into breast milk and trigger an allergy in the baby. Sometimes a mother will need to stop drinking milk and other dairy to see if this is the case. If a mother needs to go dairy-free, I would suggest she do it strictly for a week (that is, no cheese, yogurt, ice cream or milk products) than *kinda sorta* for six months. First of all, this makes it much easier to see if it works. It takes three or four days for milk to flush out of the baby. By a week, you can tell if it is making a difference. Just as important, dairy is a very good source of nutrition for a nursing mother, and if milk protein is not the culprit, she should be able to reintroduce it.

If the milk-free trial is not helpful, a close look at the rest of a mother's diet may turn up a possible culprit. Again, it is important not to make your diet unnecessarily restricted, for your own benefit. If specific foods are removed, and there is still no improvement, one option is for you to pump for a week while a trial of formula is undertaken. If the baby gets dramatically better on formula for a week, you know there is something in the breast milk that is to blame, and you go on a more detailed search to find it. One practical issue is to stay on board with breastfeeding if the formula trial works. It is completely understandable that you would want your baby to not be crying, and be tempted to stick with the formula. In most cases, though, that is not the right thing for the baby in the long term. Again, there are so many benefits of nursing that we want to only withdraw the breast milk as a last resort.

Moving on to intolerance. Intolerance of a food means that there is some component that causes unpleasant symptoms for the baby, but it is not a true allergy. A classic example would be a breastfeeding mother who eats cabbage. The baby may not like this, and may get a bellyache but it is not a true allergy. The same can certainly occur with formula. Some babies just seem to do better on one milk-based formula than another. You hear this all the time: he does great with the *Similac,* but not the *Enfamil*, or vice versa. Sometimes a different version of the exact same brand will have different ingredients- *ready-to-feed* is not identical to the powder. These are intolerances.

Lactose deserves special mention. Lactose is a sugar, which makes it a carbohydrate, not a protein. By definition, you cannot be allergic to a sugar. You can be lactose *intolerant.* Most people misunderstand this, too. Lactose intolerance is uncommon in infants. The vast majority of people who are lactose intolerant develop a problem later in childhood, or in adulthood. So, why is it that so many lactose free formulas are on the market? The answer, of course, is money. If people believe that lactose is a problem, the formula companies are more than happy to sell them this product. And if one company is cornering part of the market with a lactose free product, you can bet a competitor is going to offer it's own lactose free version. I'm sorry to say, but it is all about market share. That is not to say that some babies don't do better on the lactose free formula, but it is probably something else that is making the difference.

We used to have the same issue with iron. Some people were mistakenly convinced that iron was upsetting their baby's belly. Good medical data showed that the iron in the formula made no difference to fussiness. However, iron makes a big difference to a baby's growth and development. Fortunately, all of the popular commercial formulas now contain iron.

As you can see, it is often not that easy to figure out what part of a baby's diet is upsetting his belly. The most important thing is to look at the possible culprits one at a time, and if components of the diet are eliminated temporarily, that they be done well so a clear answer declares itself. Then Junior's biggest problem will be, "What's for dessert?"

c.   Surviving colic

A baby's cry commands immediate attention. We explain to older siblings that crying is the baby's way of letting us know that something is wrong, since they have not yet learned to talk. But what happens, as the parent, if you have tried everything- feeding, changing, burping, bouncing and whatever else you can think of, with no improvement? And what if that happens day after day and night after night? Well, that's colic.

Simply put, colic is prolonged, unexplained crying which does not have a clear cause, and which apparently is harmless to the baby. In fact, there are probably multiple conditions we don't understand that we lump together under the term colic. As new discoveries are made, all that is left is the ones we don't yet understand. For example, the baby with food allergy that we discussed earlier will likely be colicky, but this should stop once we figure out her problem and treat it.

When a baby cries and cries like this, parents usually have several concerns. The first is to make sure that nothing is seriously wrong with the baby. A visit to the doctor can usually clear this up- the typical colicky baby is well looking, and growing appropriately. The most severely affected may cry for most of her waking hours. One classic, milder pattern is the baby that cries from 5 to 11 pm (crying at this time of day is especially difficult for a parent returning home from work, who can mistakenly feel to blame). If all checks out well at the doctor's office, no tests will be ordered and reassurance will be given that the crying will go away in time. Of course, if there is a suspicion of a specific treatable cause, then that condition will become the focus. Many times, doctors will put colicky babies on diets that minimize the chance of allergy. In the same way, anti-reflux medications are prescribed, *just in case.*

The other main concern is "How do I stop the crying?" There are entire books devoted to this subject. Suffice it to say that trial and error is your best bet- swings, stroller rides, walks, *white noise* like the TV or hair dryer, car rides, baby whispering, snuggling, lullabies, and quiet are all possible helps... or not.

My biggest concern is usually the sanity of the parent(s). It is extremely difficult to hear incessant crying. It wears you down, worries you, stresses you and makes people stare at you in the grocery store. This is particularly true in difficult social situations. Lack of support, or being alone, or having low confidence about your parenting abilities or being depressed all make it tougher. While not the cause of the problem, there is no doubt that parental stress does not help it. On the other hand, in abusive situations, colic can take on a whole new level of risk. Infant colic heightens the risk of domestic and child abuse, as do other stressful situations in life.

The pediatric provider's main job, other than ensuring the baby's health, is to help the parents cope. Often, I will take the baby for a few minutes and hold him. Sometimes we get lucky and find a trick that can help a little. More often, the mother sees that he is just as fussy for me as for her, which at least helps to show that it isn't her fault. As a doctor, holding the baby gives me a whole new sensory input into the child. If she is stiff as a board no matter what I do, I get a literal feel of what they are going through (then multiplied by a thousand.)

Colic is one problem that benefits from the help of family, friends and caregivers. Volunteers to hold the baby, take her for walks or make meals all help. Emotional support from family is especially important. Parents are given permission to put the baby down for a while if nothing else is working. Most importantly, it is OK to feel like you are going crazy, and even to think bad thoughts about the baby's crying. It is essential to have a place to go or a number to call if desperate, so that a baby is never shaken, hit or harmed.

And when the colic finally goes away, at least be assured lots of colicky babies have grown up into great, happy people. You will probably never stop reminding her how much she put you through. Colic can be the ultimate test of a parent's abilities. I even tell people God must have thought you were ready to really be challenged as parents from the beginning.

Not to mention that you will want to think really hard before trying for another one. Because there is no birth control as effective as a colicky baby.

d.   There are a kabillion rules about starting solid foods

And they're all different. And they're all right, at least in someone's mind.

For new parents, starting solid food is probably the most confusing of all the tasks.

On one hand, the American Academy of Pediatrics says wait until six months of age before starting food. On the other, your baby's grandmothers might accuse you of "starving the child" if you wait longer than one month. What are you supposed to do?

The first thing to realize is that many nutrition recommendations made by doctors (not to mention friends and relatives) are not based on strong science. In fact, doctors understand food allergies about as well meteorologists understand hurricanes, which is to say, not very well. For example, in the last 20 years, we have recommended waiting to start solids to prevent children from developing food allergies. It is clear that this has not solved the food allergy problem. A recent review in the New England Journal of Medicine makes it clear: "Randomized, controlled trials of the elimination of food allergens from the diet during the first year of life or from the diet of mothers during pregnancy and breast-feeding have not shown reductions in the risk of IgE-mediated food allergies in children."(1) In fact, food allergies have become more and more common. We do know that children in developed countries are more likely to have peanut allergy than those in less developed countries. Could this be because of the way we are feeding our babies? Food additives? Industrial food processing? Time will tell, but that does not help you.

Some people would like an exact list of which food to start and when. Spoon-feeding you like that, excuse the pun, is fine if it works, but I could write the list fifty different ways. If, however, your baby does not like my list, suddenly you have a problem. And you will have a different list than your friends and relatives, which causes so much of the confusion in the first place.

Rather than a list, I prefer to give you some basic principles that can guide you while feeding, and that will work for almost everyone. Here are six rules for solids that can simply get you and your baby on a good nutritional path. It is reasonable to start at about four to six months, since there is recent evidence to suggest that waiting longer may actually *increase* the risk of developing allergies (2). In contrast, formula-fed babies given solids before four months may be at increased the risk of obesity (3).

Rule one: *listen to your baby*. You get the idea that for me this is a recurring theme. When it comes to food, listening means letting him show you when he can hold his head up well to accept (or refuse) solids. It also lets him tell you his preferences or what agrees with him. He will tell you if you made it too thick, too thin or just right. With time, he will let you know if he is hungry for a second or third daily meal when he is opening his mouth like a little bird. If he spits it away or fusses, he probably does not want it. Many people will first try to introduce a second daily meal a month or so after starting solids, but that is just a guide.

Rule two: be mindful of *allergic* foods. To be honest, the rules here are all going to change in the next couple of years. While we used to say leave the most *allergic foods* for last, there is brand new evidence to say that waiting too long to introduce certain foods increases a baby's risk of food allergy (4). Doctors are only just beginning to get their heads around this information, but it is clear that there will soon be a major shift in the way babies are fed. For now, when a sibling or parent food allergies, or the baby has a suggestion of serious risk for allergy (such as severe eczema), introducing solids under the supervision of an allergist may be the way to go.

Here is one important and underemphasized point: *the most likely allergic food for your baby is the one to which your family members have been allergic.* Everything else is based on the odds that a food will cause allergies in the overall population, which is much less specific. If no one in the family has allergies, this is a good thing. Your baby will probably not have an issue. Most people will still start with baby cereal, fruit or vegetable. Of course, this doesn't mean that you give your baby a peanut butter, strawberry, crab omelet on the same day! One food at a time still makes sense.

Milk allergy is a little different than most people think. Milk is a common allergy, but we give it to newborns, since most women have dairy in their diet when they nurse, and most regular formulas are *cow's milk based*. So, it is not necessary to withhold all dairy products until age one. The reason we recommend waiting to switch to (whole) cow's milk as a main nutritional source has to do with other nutrients, especially iron, which is low in cow's milk, and is poorly-absorbed. In other words, a little yogurt here and there in the second half of the first year is not a problem.

Rule three: introduce *one new food at a time*. For convenience, we say wait half a week to a week before adding the next food. This way, if green beans go right through him, or if rice cereal causes constipation, you know. Of course, you can wait longer than this between foods if you want, especially at the beginning.

Rule four: *no honey* in the first year. Honey can cause botulism in infants (5). Unlike in older children and adults, infant botulism can lead to temporary paralysis, including the need for a respirator to breathe. I don't know why babies are more susceptible, they just are.

Rule five: table food (what everyone else is eating) is for *when the baby can sit in the high chair at the table* and start to feed himself. Finger foods usually start with something like *Cheerios* or puffs. Healthy babies older than six months with normal swallowing rarely have trouble handling these textures. Sitting at the high chair serves the dual purpose of keeping the baby still and safe. Remember, many young children choke when food is combined with motion.

Rule six: *no Nacho chips.* This is my way of saying to be careful about texture. Early solids are soft and do not require chewing. As teeth come in and the baby does well with a soft diet, you can progress to firmer textures, but clearly choking foods should be avoided. A choking food is anything that could block the baby's airway if swallowed whole. Grapes, nuts and pieces of hot dog are common examples. And Nacho chips- even during the Super Bowl.

e.   Constipation is a state of poop, not a state of calendar

"Call Mrs. Jones. Scarlett has had no bowel movement since Friday."

At least weekly, there is a message like this on my desk. In all likelihood, a similar message is on the desk of every primary care provider in the country. I always smile and think back to the Rowe family, my childhood neighbors. Their bathroom had a wall hanging which described an argument between the body's organs. They all claimed to be the most important. The bowels went last, and after that, no one argued anymore.

Constipation is miserable, especially for little kids. Before we talk about prevention and treatment, it is very important to understand normal bowel function. After birth (and occasionally before), a baby will pass the stool which has been formed while the baby is still inside her mother. This *meconium* is well known to any parent who has changed one of baby's first diapers. It is thick, tarry, messy, and probably represents one of Mother Nature's best tricks on new parents. The first diapers you change are definitely the most difficult. *Failure to pass meconium within 48 hours after birth is a red flag that there is a problem.* When the meconium has finished passing, the stool temporarily becomes a green color, which is known as transitional stool because it only lasts for a couple of days. Infrequent stooling in the first week sometimes suggests that the baby is not getting enough to eat.

After the first few days, normal depends on what she is drinking. Breast-milk poop is classically called mustard-seed yellow, a description you will understand once you see it. It is very loose and at times can take on almost a watery consistency, which is lovely when it goes straight up Scarlett's back and ruins her entire outfit for the day. Babies feeding only on breast milk seldom if ever get constipated. Breast-fed babies often poop after every feeding early on.

Sometimes it will take a while for a young baby get the poop out. This could be ten minutes or most of the day. I think of this as bowel immaturity- essentially, the bowel has not yet become coordinated enough to be efficient, and the contractions in the bowel are not that effective. As long as the baby is doing otherwise all right, this is usually normal.

Within a few weeks something interesting happens- babies either continue to poop this often or they don't. I usually quote a *normal frequency of breast fed bowel movements of between ten per day and once every ten days*. This is a huge range, but it can actually be broader than that. I talked to one pediatrician who had a breastfed baby who went an entire month without a bowel movement. It is a testament to just how efficiently breast milk can be absorbed. This was a normal, healthy baby who was happy, growing and did not have a bloated belly, which are the key questions to ask before assuming that everything is all right.

Formula-fed babies are somewhat more predictable. The *normal range for formula poop is about four times per day to once every four days*. Formula stool tends to be firmer than breast poop, and constipation can occur. There are multiple infant formulas on the market, and so there is no one formula poop. Some give looser stools than others. Soy is well known for its tendency to constipate certain children. If constipation develops, your provider will be able to help with suggestions for easier products to pass.

Stool color is another thing over which you can spare yourself worry. With apologies to my gastroenterologist friends for oversimplifying it, poop color is not that complicated. When food

99

hits the bowel, the gall bladder contracts. The gall bladder is a small sac under the liver which stores *bile*, and this bile is the green stuff that gives stool its color. More bile means more green, so the color of stool really depends on how much the gall bladder felt like squeezing. I am not concerned about which part of the yellow-green-brown paint palate wins out in Scarlett's diaper on a particular day. Doctors really only care about three colors: black stool (with the exception of newborn meconium) can reflect old blood in the bowel, and red stool can reflect fresh blood, both of which are abnormal. White stool suggests the complete absence of bile, which is also a concern. By the way, *green vomit* is a totally different story- this *can indicate a blockage or obstruction should prompt immediate medical follow-up.*

All righty then. We have the scoop on normal poop. Now, let's discuss constipation, which is practically defined as stool which is hard and uncomfortable to pass. Stool can build up in the colon, leading to more discomfort. It can begin in infancy for formula-fed babies and after the introduction of baby food for breast-fed babies. Like most other conditions, it will be a combination of genetics and environment: in this case, the child being prone to it, as well as her intake. There are varying severities, of course, ranging from extra time and discomfort having a bowel movement, right up to passage of blood from straining, belly bloating, poor feeding and general misery.

Since we can't change a baby's natural predisposition, we treat constipation by adjusting the diet. As I mentioned above, if the baby is only on formula, a formula change may help. Sometimes, even this can be avoided with little tricks. If the baby is growing well, and especially if she is chubby, 2 to 4 ounces of water per day can provide a little bit of extra stool softness. Various other products including prune juice, and apricot nectar, used sparingly, can also help a lot. This can be a teaspoon added to each bottle, or up to 2 ounces diluted with the same amount of water once/day. The goal is an easy bowel movement about once or twice per day.

Once solids are introduced, these can also be used to the baby's advantage. For cereals, rice tends to be the most constipating, followed by oatmeal, followed by barley. A change from rice to barley cereal can really help. In the same way, bananas, applesauce, and orange vegetables are generally felt to slow the bowels, while peaches, prunes, and greens speed them up. A little experimentation is usually all that is needed.

If diet alone doesn't help, medicines are sometimes necessary. For short-term relief of a very fussy baby, a suppository of glycerin will usually help. Taking the temperature with a rectal thermometer will usually have the same effect. We try to avoid stronger medications in the first year of life. For older children with recurrent constipation, medicine by mouth is preferred. Many medications are on the market, which all have their pros and cons. Here are a few brief words about one to avoid, and one to look for. Mineral oil was used a lot in the past for older children. It should not be used for infants under 1 year, since infants tend to throw up a lot, and the oil can be aspirated into the lungs. The problem with almost all the older medicines is taste. More and more these days, we go straight to polyethylene glycol (PEG), which has been marketed under the name *Miralax*. The great thing about PEG is that it has been made into a tasteless powder, which can be dissolved in other liquids. It is now used extensively, and is available over the counter.

Parents are often concerned about potential adverse effects of the long-term use of bowel medicines. Doctors are a lot less concerned. PEG is not addictive in any way and does not interfere with the body's natural function. As one gastroenterologist I know put it, driving through traffic for an hour into the city to talk to a specialist about PEG is significantly more dangerous than using this product for an extended period of time.

For how long should PEG be used? It depends on how long the problem has been present. A good rule of thumb is to use the medicine for as long as the constipation has been present. Constipation for a week can be treated for a week. Chronic constipation should be treated for at least three months. This is because the rectum of a chronically constipated child stretches to make room for the extra poop. Even when the cleanout has been completed, it takes a long time for this stretched bowel to relax down to normal size and regain the elastic properties that help normal bowel movements to occur.

As Scarlett gets older, the constipation may or may not improve. The diet tends to change significantly in the second year and beyond. This can be for better or worse. Cheese, the great constipator, starts to make its way into the diet of many kids at this time. Mac and cheese, pizza and the other staples of picky eaters need to be limited. On the upside, if vegetables and fiber can be introduced, bowel movements may become easier. Greater activity levels also help to promote pooping, as does the ability to assume the squatting position.

As the age of toilet-training approaches, a big kid can be taught to sit on the potty for a few minutes after a mealtime. This takes advantage of the *gastro-colic reflex*, which is essentially *something in, something out*, and is the reason why newborns go so often. The body naturally *wants* the bowels to move about 15 minutes after eating, making this the ideal time to toilet. Sitting in a way that the feet are flat on the floor helps to make use of the child's abdominal muscles. A low-to-the-ground potty helps this, as will a footstool next to a regular toilet.

Constipation during toilet training can be an absolute non-starter. Constipated adults will think to themselves, "I know it's going to hurt, but I have to go." By contrast, kids will think, "It hurts, so I'm not going." In other words, "A child in pain, ain't gonna train." This can lead to a fear of the potty, a holding on cycle and multiple frustrations for child and parents. The best way to avoid the frustration (other than diffusing any pressure from adults) is to make sure that pooping is easy and non painful. In other words, toilet training time is not the time to stop the bowel medication.

Dr. Garrett Zella, one of my gastroenterologist mentors, likes to make the point that kids should be rewarded for *sitting* on the potty, rather than for successfully pooping. For a constipated kid, just sitting down there can provoke anxiety. There can be a fear of pain and a fear of failure. If the reward is only for poop, then the child can easily become discouraged. On the other hand, kids who get praised for sitting control their own destiny.

As a child gets older, parents of constipated kids often ask, "Shouldn't we be able to stop the medicine by now?" My answer is that if you want to change what comes out, you have to change what goes in! In other words, if a high fiber diet with lots of fluids can be achieved, the need for medicine will go down. Until that time, medication is likely to remain necessary.

I guess that bathroom wall hanging got it right. The bowels are the bosses of the body.

f.   With the tummy bug, the tortoise beats the hare

There's not much worse than throwing up. Except perhaps when your child does it. When a young child has vomiting and diarrhea, the poor thing doesn't even understand what is happening to his body. As if just feeling that bad wasn't enough. You want them to feel better as soon as possible. You definitely want them to stay out of the hospital emergency room. A slow but steady approach is your best bet.

Every illness is different, as is each vomiting and diarrhea bug, but most tend to start with feeling nauseous, followed by some amount of vomiting. Often times it is fast and furious at first, with a short period of time after throwing up where you feel a little bit better until the next wave comes. If the vomiting is coming more often than every hour, there is not much point in fighting it. Whatever goes down will just come back up again. With any luck this doesn't last too long.

Once the vomiting slows down, you can try giving him a sip. For nursing mothers, a minute on the breast is plenty. For other kids, we usually start with a teaspoon to a one half ounce to drink. The ideal fluid to give is an *oral electrolyte solution*, the best known of which is *Pedialyte*. The reason that we like these drinks is that they contain the right balance of salt, sugar and water. Plain water has no nutrients. Juice, soda and sports drinks have too much sugar, which can promote diarrhea. Many kids, especially older ones, will fight taking electrolyte solutions- they don't taste the greatest. Making them cold helps. You can buy oral electrolyte popsicles, but you can also just make your own slushies by not quite freezing the drink. If nothing else works, a splash of a better tasting liquid can sometimes help, but resist the temptation to dilute the good effects of the electrolyte solution, which was designed to best hydrate your child.

If a sip to a half ounce stays down, keep doing this every 15 to 20 minutes. You can set the microwave timer to let him know when it is OK to drink again. Repeat this for an hour or two and then *slowly* increase how much you are giving. You can then begin to space out the time to every 30 to 60 minutes. Remember, slow and steady is what works. Most kids are really thirsty and want to drink more than they can stomach. Many parents feel bad for their kids or rush to get them rehydrated. This usually ends with throwing up again. If this happens, wait an hour and then try again from the beginning. It will usually work.

Contrary to what many people think, milk is a really good fluid to rehydrate. Breast milk certainly is. So is infant formula. For children who are over a year of age, cow's milk can be tried as soon as the electrolyte solution is staying down consistently. Again, if it comes back up, retreat to the electrolyte solution for a while. There are two things to know about milk. First, it will prolong the diarrhea somewhat, but your child will *feel better* sooner because of the calories and nutrition in the milk. Second, if diarrhea has been going strong for several days, the bowels may temporarily lose what they need to break down and absorb lactose, the milk sugar. In this case, milk, which is lactose-free, such as soy milk, is a better temporary choice.

Diarrhea usually begins after the vomiting, as the illness makes its way down the pipe. The good news is that if vomiting stops, and fluids can be kept down, diarrhea on its own will usually not dehydrate a child unless it is severe. As we mentioned earlier, breast-fed infants often have in excess of ten bowel movements a day, but still grow just fine. It is the vomiting that is usually what gets you.

It is important to know when to call the doctor. *Green or bloody vomit, and bloody diarrhea* are obvious concerns. With dehydration, the lips and tears will start to become dry. Wet diapers will go down- a little bit is just a sign that the body is adapting, but *no wet diapers for more than 12 hours* is usually not a good sign. Most kids will not have much energy with this illness, but a change from *couch potato* to *wet noodle* is not good. *Frequent vomiting that lasts* more than 24 hours in a young baby, and 48 hours in an older child is not great either. If in doubt, call.

Fortunately most of these illnesses are short-lived, and there is nothing better than not feeling nauseous and really enjoying a meal again.

Oh, and get your infant the rotavirus immunization. This dramatically reduces the chance of hospitalization from the worst of the stomach viruses.

g. Beware of the child with vomiting but no diarrhea

This is what doctors call a truism. I learned it as a medical student from the Chief of Pediatrics, Dr. Jim Boone. He told me he learned it from his Chief of Pediatrics. It was true 60 years ago and it is still true today. The reason is simple: vomiting and diarrhea is the stomach bug 99 times out of 100- not pleasant, but usually brief and not serious. Vomiting without diarrhea on the other hand can be anything from soup to nuts, or head to guts as it were.

The explanation is complicated, but I will try to explain it clearly. When we are sick, the body has a limited number of things that it can do to protest. Some of these are particular to the part of the body affected- cough for the head and chest, for example. There are a few symptoms that are shared by many parts of the body - fever, loss of appetite, fatigue and vomiting are some of the most basic. Of these, vomiting is the one that fools people because they mistakenly assume that vomiting is always a belly problem. While serious belly problems usually include vomiting in their symptoms, serious problems elsewhere in the body can also have vomiting with the main symptom. These include infections of the kidney (urinary tract), and spinal column (meningitis), which will usually cause a fever, too. Pneumonia can occasionally occur with fever and vomiting, sometimes even without a cough. Vomiting without fever can occur with bowel obstruction (blockages), inflammation of the pancreas, and even increased pressure on the brain.

My main concern writing this passage is to keep you from becoming too anxious every time your child throws up, but still educating you on the potential concerns. It is an important enough topic to be worth the effort. For doctors and for parents, this is a classic example of *don't assume*. All you need to do, as a parent, is to watch your child and keep your provider informed. The rest is up to the provider's office. If you are concerned about a serious problem, persistent vomiting without diarrhea is a time you may have to insist for a visit if your call is brushed off.

Although it is more the doctor's job to diagnose specific problems, here are some serious symptoms about which you should call. It is worth repeating that *green or bloody vomit* is not OK, nor is *blood in the stool*. Periods of severe crying with apparent normal periods in between can suggest a blockage that is coming and going. *Repeated nighttime vomiting or vomiting immediately on wakening* can be a sign of raised brain pressure. Symptoms suggestive of a specific problem elsewhere, such as *foul smelling urine* in a kidney infection should always be reported. Remember, this is simply a guide. Your care provider will advise you best about your child.

h.   Calories consumed minus calories used equals calories gained

It is a shockingly simple formula, with which we continue to struggle.

I want to start by saying that twenty years ago I would not have included a calorie intake chapter in a book for young children. The general thought was that if obesity was a problem, age 7 was a good time to deal with it, because kids, by then, would have safely outgrown their baby fat. In some ways, this was based on the knowledge that age 6 is roughly the skinniest of our life, which is a useful general principal, both for reassuring parents of skinny kids, and for making a point about overweight kids.

As we all know, obesity rates have skyrocketed. For this reason, this discussion routinely begins at about age 2 years. This is over and above the routine nutrition discussions that occur for all families. Unfortunately, it is not unusual to need to discuss obesity at 15 to 18 months for heavy kids, and in fact, occasionally I do it in the first year, when there is an obvious issue with food choices and quantities. Think for a minute just how awful it is to have to tell parents that their beautiful baby is on his way to serious obesity.

With that backdrop, let's talk numbers.

If I eat and drink more than I use, I will gain calories. If I eat and drink less than I use, I will lose calories. Calories measure energy, and so gained calories means extra energy. This energy is stored in our body's fat cells. In other words, gained calories means gained weight.

You will see that I have not mentioned what *kind* of food is being consumed. 100 calories of protein has the same energy as 100 calories of fat or 100 calories of carbs. A calorie is a calorie is a calorie. This *does not at all mean* that all foods have equal nutrition. It just means that if weight loss is the issue, the calories consumed are what matters. So, whether it is high protein, low carb, low fat or high rhubarb, if you know the calories consumed, you know what is important. If you want to know how many calories are in a serving of anything, this can readily be found on packages, or on the Internet- you can even scan bar codes to get your information. These days you can get apps that will help promote healthy weight and lifestyle. Many apps can track calorie intake and use, although applying research-tested pediatric goals to these apps is still in its early days.

Do you need to count calories for your overweight child? This is the most logical option. Nutritionists do this, and they will recommend that a certain number of calories be consumed each day, depending on the child's weight, height, and calorie use. If you are a numbers person, this is a good idea. It is also time-consuming.

An easier, but less precise option is to simply reduce the calories by removing unnecessary intake. For example, you can begin by taking away all snack foods, especially crackers, cookies and bars. Clearly, no snack is less than whatever was in the snack. If you remove all soda and juice, and have water in its place, that is also a switch to a zero calorie option. In the same way, if you reduce a portion size, you will make a definite improvement, although the exact amount may be less clear.

The proof in the pudding (or lack of pudding) is the results you achieve. In other words, if your child's weight is moving towards the goal, your changes are working. If not, you need to do more.

But what should be your goal? For young children, it may not be for weight loss at all. We often encourage *growing into her weight*, because by keeping the weight the same, she will slim out as she grows. You will have a certain target weight or calorie intake in your mind. *There is no need to share that with a child.* I would also discourage frequent weigh-ins; in fact, you are probably better off not weighing him at all at home. Focus on healthy eating (portions and choices) for your family. This will get results and preserve self-esteem. Remember that *modeling* good behavior is very important, both in terms of parents making good nutrition choices and in terms of not being obsessed with the weigh scale or the mirror. Rather than, "Don't eat that because you are too heavy (or worse yet, *fat*)", the emphasis is, "We eat this (or don't eat that) because it is (or is not) good for us."

Activity and electronics use play key roles in the other side of the equation; that is, in the *calories used*. Reductions in activity and increases in electronics use have also contributed to our obesity problem. It is ironic that while I am talking to a parent about their child's weight issue, the child is commonly watching a video or playing on the parents phone. For years, pediatricians have recognized the connection between electronic media consumption and obesity. We are certainly losing that battle currently, as technology increasingly brings screens into our every moment. I find myself increasingly taking the hard line by telling parents to remove all screens from their young child's world. While few are able to achieve this goal, it at least sends a clear message.

Activity is another key, and one where most parents have a hard time setting a good example. My choice of the word activity is important. It does not have to be organized, and it definitely does not need to be sports. It begins with stroller rides in infancy, progresses to walks and exploring and, of course, should mainly evolve into play. There is nothing like a good game of tag.

In all of these areas- intake, activity and electronics- three things are important. The first is to pick goals that are achievable and that are easy to maintain. Cutting out the foods that no one would miss is a simple example of this. The second is support, whether from your doctor, a friend or both. It is clear that few people can do it alone. The third is regular follow-up. By checking in with your care provider, you can monitor progress, get feedback, tips and revise both calories consumed and calories used.

This is a really challenging problem. It is one of the toughest. The good news is that you have time on your side and the most important motivator in the world- the health of those two eyes looking up at you. They can help both of you get to a healthier place.

Just do the math!

i.   Picking your battles with picky eaters

Some people eat to live and some people live to eat. This statement is as true of children as it is of adults. Feeding a picky eater is a source of great frustration for many parents. Most of this frustration can be relieved with a brief crash course in nutrition.

Toddler eating is a fascinating subject to think about, and a fun one to watch, except perhaps when you are the parent. A toddler is an eater in transition. Most babies have initially been allowed to drink whenever they wanted. As solids were introduced, there starts to be a variety in both what is being served and how often it is served. The majority of parents are relatively easy-going in their expectations of what an infant will eat in his first year. After that first birthday, however, many parents feel a pressure that their children should start eating three meals per day. The truth is that most toddlers eat one good, one bad and one in between meal per day. Some seem to live off their baby fat like bears in hibernation, and hardly eat at all as toddlers. Others convince their parents that it is time to shift their savings from the college fund to the second fridge fund.

Take home message number one: *Do not stress if your child does not eat his dinner.*

There is nothing like a bad dinner for a good breakfast the next morning. You might feel awful putting him to bed without eating, but once you realize that it is not worth trying to feed someone that is not hungry, you will feel better. It is unusual for a healthy child to be deficient in calories, provided the food is available to be offered. Offering three meals a day is appropriate for a parent. Deciding which ones to eat is appropriate for a child. If you have concerns that your child is truly lacking in calories, ask your care provider.

There are some young children who do not gain weight well. Remember our formula from the last chapter: calories consumed minus calories used equals calories gained. We used this to discuss obesity, but can use it to understand slow weight gain. If a baby is not gaining weight, he may not be consuming enough calories. Sometimes the calories are consumed, but the body has trouble absorbing them. This occurs when there is an issue with the bowels, such as severe allergy or intolerance of certain foods such as gluten (known as Celiac Disease). Finally, if the body is using extra calories, which can happen with breathing and heart conditions, the intake may not be enough to keep up with demand. Almost all of these babies will look or act sick in some way, depending on the problem. They will also have growth curves that do not look normal. Some of us are big and others are small, but steady growth at a certain speed over time is what we look for.

Pediatricians love growth curves, because they are just a great way to monitor health. If a child is maintaining growth at a steady speed, there is a very good chance that he is healthy. When the growth drops off, a closer look is in order. A happy toddler with normal energy, normal bowel patterns and otherwise good health is probably going to end up fine, especially when her size is following siblings or parents. This is especially true for a chubby baby who is not meant to be a chubby older child. In the old days, this was called losing your baby fat. When it is unclear whether a problem truly exists, we do lab tests to make sure.

An increase in calories for underweight children is occasionally recommended. We do this by eliminating juice, which results in more milk and better solid intake, as well as by calorie boosting. Calorie boosting is accomplished by adding butter to mashed potatoes, cheese to vegetables, and peanut butter to toast- in other words, adding fats/oils. I always have some cautiousness about overdoing the supplements. The first caution is that we do not want you to become too obsessed with your child's intake. Obsessing over food increases stress for you and your child. It also can sow the seeds for eating disorders down the road. From a medical perspective, some children are converted from eating very healthy, vegetable rich diets, to ones that are higher in animal fats. These fats are not good for us, as we get older, since they increase the risk of heart disease. There is also some evidence to suggest that babies who are born *small for gestational age,* that is, less than 5 ½ pounds at full term, are already at a higher risk for diabetes in later life. The reasons for this are not clear, but I do wonder whether overfeeding in an attempt to catch up is harmful in the long run.

For toddlers who are growing normally, focus on iron and nutrients, not protein. In North America, as long as enough food is offered, protein deficiency is uncommon. According to the Academy of Nutrition and Dietetics, "while children's intakes of solid fats and added sugars exceed guidelines, many are not meeting the recommended intake for the nutrients of public health concern (calcium, dietary fiber, potassium, and vitamin D), whole grains, vegetables, fruits, and dairy foods." *Iron deficiency* is rampant. Many kids are poor at getting iron-rich food. Some do not like red meat (ham is most palatable for most toddlers). As a North American society, adults are poor at offering non-meat sources of iron. Think about beans, greens, and iron-fortified cereals- a quick look at the side of a box will tell you about the iron in the latter. Keep in mind that toddlers who drink more than four servings of milk per day are also at risk for low iron. Young children are screened for iron deficiency yearly at well visits.

117

Take home message number two: *offer vegetables that are high in iron.*

As mentioned above, vitamins and other minerals are also hard to come by for children. Now, I admit to having a fifteen-year-old who has yet to befriend a green vegetable except lettuce, and I understand that you can offer, but you cannot (and should not) force them to eat it. Modeling good vegetable behavior by parents will help in the long run. For picky kids, sometimes the best thing to do is to invite their curiosity by having the vegetables on your plate. I tell kids that Mother Nature made it easy by color-coding the vegetables- we should eat red, orange, yellow and green ones. Again, many cereals are also fortified with vitamins and minerals. Some parents have the skill to get creative with blenders and even sneak things into baked goods. If you do not, that is why vitamin supplements were invented.

Take home message number three: *get color on your plates.*

There is another advantage of real fruits and vegetables. We are just beginning to learn about some of the other beneficial substances that they contain. These include foods such as avocado, blueberries and other dark berries, and spinach. These foods contain what we call anti-oxidants, which are natural substances that reduce harmful chemicals known as free radicals. Free radicals are involved in inflammation and cancer, among other things. As a result, antioxidants have come to be known as *super foods*. Many of them actually taste good, too!

Take home message number four: *supercharge her diet with super foods.*

The biggest downfall of the North American diet (other than the amount we eat) is our consumption of animal fat. Most recommendations suggest that fat make up 30 to 40 percent of calories for children 3 and under, and 20 to 35 per cent of older children and adults. Not all fats are created equal. The terms animal fat and saturated fat are often incorrectly used interchangeably. As with most things, the more we learn, the more complicated it gets. Saturated fats from animals are generally felt to be less healthy, whereas saturated fats from vegetable sources may be healthier. You will also hear about *trans* fats, which can occur in animal products, but more often are created in processed foods. Trans fats and saturated animal fats raise the unhealthy cholesterol levels in the body, which increase the risk for heart disease. We know that heart disease is life-long in the making, so it does actually matter how our children eat. More importantly, we become used to the foods we are exposed to in our childhood.

You may have heard of the Mediterranean diet. Researchers over the last 50 years have become aware that something about the way Southern Europeans eat is better than how we do it. The types of oil used are key. Vegetable oils, especially olive oil, are a much healthier source of fat than animal fat. Fish oils are also higher in these *unsaturated* fats. Entire books have been written on various types of olive oil, but here are a couple of interesting things: the more *virgin*, the better, and *light* usually means more processed, not lower calorie.

Take home message number four: *discover olive oil.*

I have to take a brief moment to discuss *organic* foods. Many people are misled in this regard. As you probably know, *organic* is a term that refers to the way that a product was raised, and usually refers to avoiding certain chemicals in the production of the food. However, there is very little regulation of what this word means. If organic means locally raised and an avoidance of pesticides, it makes sense for the environment. There is not a lot of evidence that most organic foods are better for your child. It seems like a good idea to avoid routinely giving antibiotics to livestock. Things like organic formula bother me, because they seem to be just another manipulation of parents to buy a certain product. As we all know, organic is synonymous with expensive.

Take home message number five*: be skeptically organic.*

Finally, it is common to hear people discuss the cost of healthy foods. This is undoubtedly true. As one grandmother told me, "I can make a whole tray of American Chop Suey for the cost of one meal of fish." I totally get this, but there are ways you can optimize quality at low cost. Many of you are much better than me at shopping sales and stocking up. Eating *in season* local fruits and vegetables usually increases quality and decreases price. Most of all, serve smaller portions to adults and older kids. It always costs less to eat less. Whole grain products are more filling. Don't buy crap.

Take home message number six: *less is more.*

j.   It is worth finding religion about your baby's teeth

"When should my child see the dentist?"

We used to say age 3. Now, pediatric dentists say age 1. A horrific number of cavities can occur by age 3, and many children with cavities require general anesthetics to remove or repair the rotten teeth. When surgery is required, we have all failed- the community, for not having fluoridated water; the pediatrician for not teaching good early dental care; and the parent, for not carrying it out. So, the better question is, "How can I help my child have good teeth?" With this approach, the dentist will be happy, regardless.

Babies usually get first teeth between 4 and 12 months of age, starting with the *incisor*s in the middle. The first set finishes with the second molars, sometime after the second birthday. In total, young kids get 20 teeth. The order and timing can vary. Some kids suffer through every one; with others, you only know when you look. People argue about whether teething can cause fever, but a fever of 101 or higher is unlikely to be from teething.

A few simple steps can result in a very good set of teeth 99 percent of the time. Here they are:
   1.   Brush the teeth as soon as they come in. A finger brush or cloth works fine, too. You do not need fluoride toothpaste until age two, and even then, just a pea-size portion will do,

since kids tend to swallow most of it. Brushing twice per day is preferable.

2. Learn whether or not your town has fluoridated water. If not, your provider will recommend giving fluoride drops beginning at 6 months.

3. Wean pre-bed feedings as early as is practical, and definitely by a year of age. This includes breast milk, formula, and cow's milk- all contain sugar. It is fine to feed the baby in the evening, but you want to brush the teeth afterwards. You want to avoid having her fall asleep on the bottle, breast or cup. The same goes for the middle of the night. If you find this difficult to accomplish, a bedtime feeding of water can buy you time.

4. Avoid juice. Four ounces of apple juice has 13-14 grams of sugar (1,2), so even if watered down, there is still a lot of sugar. The only kids for whom I recommend juice are the constipated ones. If you need juice for this reason, give it all at one time, and not right before sleep.

5. Do not allow your toddler to sip her cup or bottle through the day. The amount of time that sugar contacts the teeth is very important. In other words, if she has a sip of her drink every 30 minutes, there is always sugar in the mouth, like a hard candy. As an aside, tripping with a cup in the mouth is also a common way to injure the mouth.

6. Wean the pacifier and bottle by age 12 months. These goals can be as hard as quitting smoking for adults. You need to plan ahead, and know it will be a rough few days. A child

will drink from a cup before she dehydrates herself, I promise. I do not live in your house to know when life permits this stress, but I do know that a bottle to a twelve-month-old is a nutritional source, while to an eighteen-month-old, it is a security blanket. Thumbs are harder, and generally require her cooperation, which will not be practical until about age 4.

7. Know risk factors which would make your child at risk for dental disease. These include stomach reflux (due to the effect of acid on the teeth), frequent antibiotic use and difficulty with carrying out steps 1-6.

Dentists can stop the progression of caries or pre-caries states with an early visit. There are dental applications that can strengthen the teeth if used early. My experience is that dentists are also better *bad cops* than pediatricians, for parents who need to be read the riot act.

A final word about brushing. Recognize that even the most independent toddler cannot brush her teeth alone. Let her brush if she wants, but you need to brush afterwards. If brushing results in a nuclear tantrum, sit down on the ground and make a *V* with your legs. Put her head in the point of the *V*. Restrain her legs with yours, and her arms if needs be. This allows you to use one hand to open her mouth and the other one to brush. You won't need to do this many times- she will soon let you brush rather than be put through the torture.

We all want good teeth for our children. Even more so, parents feel tremendous guilt when bad caries develop. It is common for them to say that they wish they knew.

Well, now you know.

k. Boys might never fully toilet train, if not for girls

Think about the guys you know. They're watching the big game-cold drink in one hand and snack in the other. Do they plan to get up at halftime, or just put on the diaper and change later? I am willing to bet at least some would choose the latter. Toilet training occurs earlier on Venus than on Mars.

As we discuss elsewhere, not all boys are from Mars nor are all girls from Venus. However, if your child is Martian, and is taking his/her sweet time with the process, this may give you some consolation. And when great grandma says that she would have had Junior trained "by now", she is probably right. Forty years ago, kids began toilet training several months earlier than they do now (1). How much of that is different pressures and expectations, and how much of it is more comfortable diapers, I'm not sure.

If my goal in this book is to give you tips that aren't found elsewhere, then this chapter should be brief. There are *plenty* of good resources on toilet training and there is more than one way to

124

do it. Here are just a few thoughts that might be useful. The goal is to make it a positive experience for everyone involved.

Toilet training should begin when the child is developmentally ready. The two most common techniques to train a child require different levels of maturity. A minority of people use *parent driven* training. This involves sitting the child on the potty routinely several times a day, especially after meals/drinks, when the child is more likely to have to go anyway. Since the parent determines the cues, the child can be less mature when starting, This is typically in the second year, although in some cultures it begins in early infancy. Most kids are trained when the child is ready- the child senses the cues and the parent guides them on what to do. Since it is *child driven*, the child has to be more mature, typically at least 18 months. Think about where your child is at with other development skills to take away some of the pressure. For example, if your two-year-old is slower in walking, talking, and social skills, this can be a clue that it is too early to toilet train.

The second tip is to make sure that he is pooping easily before trying to bowel train. As I said before, "a child in pain, ain't gonna train." You will know if constipation is a problem for him. Modify his diet and use medication if necessary to make toileting easy. This will remove a huge amount of grief and frustration for everyone involved. Constipation-prone kids probably train better with a kid's potty on the floor than a ring in the adult toilet, because they can plant their feet on the ground and get better leverage.

I am not aware of any research on pull-ups, but intuitively they don't make sense. Part of the reward of toilet training is the comfort of wearing big kid underwear. If you don't have to earn that feeling, you lose part of the incentive. And they cost more. I suppose the rare kid who did NOT like underwear could be trained first to pull-ups.

Do not routinely use pre-school as a carrot to encourage toilet training because it can backfire. Preschool is a big transition in itself. Even a child who seems to want to go might be nervous inside. You might sabotage both by tying the two together- in other words, the toileting ends up going slower because of pre-school anxiety.

Some kids really resist pooping on the toilet. Everyone knows this guy because he hides when it is time for a bowel movement. Older preschoolers sometimes ask for a diaper just to poop. Whatever the reason, it can be helped by a gradual technique. First, allow him the diaper, but encourage the bathroom as the hiding place. After a time, have him sit on the potty in a diaper. Next, open the diaper on the potty. Then, remove the diaper.

One last point: nighttime dryness has nothing to do with the rest of toilet training. At night, the bladder is the alarm clock, and the brain has to hear it. If the alarm clock isn't loud enough, you sleep through it. Kids who are wet at night can generally sleep through a bomb. If you have ever tried to bring this boy to the bathroom at midnight, it is like carrying a sack of potatoes. It will improve with time, when the body is ready, although there are good alarm techniques and medicines for older kids. I always remember, "seven percent of seven-year-olds" are wet at night. Most of them are boys. Put another way, in every second grade class, two boys are still wet at night; they almost certainly do not know each other's identity. Make sure your child with nighttime wetting knows it is not his fault, and it will get better in time.

As for daytime bladder training for boys, I really would like to invent a potty that looks like a tree.

l.   Noshakiditis and other issues with private parts

Once every week or two, a mother will bring her son in to check for a possible bladder infection. Typically, he will be 4 or 5 years old, and will have begun having burning in his penis when he pees. With few exceptions, I know before going in the room that the problem is *noshakiditis*.

When a boy or man finishes going pee, there is usually a small amount of urine that remains in the penis. For this reason, when boys learn to pee standing up, they should be taught to gently shake the tip of the penis for a second or two after voiding. This releases those last few drop from the penis. If they do not, the pee will eventually drip into the underwear. The tip of the penis will be in contact with the damp underwear, leading to an irritation. This is what usually causes the inflammation and burning. We call inflamed tonsils tonsillitis, and an inflamed appendix is called appendicitis. If you do not shake your pee-pee, I call the resulting inflammation no-*shake-it-itis*, or, noshakiditis.

Noshakiditis occurs in circumcised and uncircumcised boys. In uncircumcised boys, the urine can pool in the end of the foreskin. Either way, the opening of the penis, called the urethral meatus, is a little irritated. Urine is not the only irritant that causes noshakiditis. Water in a wet swimsuit and bubbles in the tub can be equally irritating. A new laundry detergent or even sweaty pajamas can occasionally do the same thing.

Noshakiditis can also cause a feeling of having to go urgently. In little boys, this will inevitably lead to urinary accidents. Most annoying for parents is when Johnny wants to go pee literally every five minutes. Although he feeds like he has to go, most of the time it is just that the irritation is giving him this sensation. Usually, only a few drops come out. Some parents will be aware that diabetes often shows up with frequent urination. The difference is that, in diabetes, there is a large volume of urine each time.

Girls are also prone to irritation. For them, incorrect wiping is often the culprit. Most people try to teach girls to wipe front to back. In my experience, this is a potty pipe dream. You can correct me if I am wrong, but my guess is that most adult women do not even do this unless they are either anoretentive or have a history of bladder infections. Instead, most little girls will wait to last minute, run to the bathroom, pee, quickly go woosh-woosh-woosh with the paper in a back and forth motion, then run back to play. Hopefully, they stop first to flush and wash their hands.

Here is an attempt at a remedy for the wiping problem. I make the assumption that little girls will not consistently remember the correct direction to wipe and recognize that wiping itself is irritating. Instead, I explain that after a girl pees, the job of the paper is to make sure that her private area is dry. You have to hold the paper on the private area long enough for all the wetness to go on the paper. Slowly counting to five does the trick. Girls who are toilet-trained can almost always do this. In fact, even older girls often get a kick out of slowly counting like they were just learning to count again.

For boys, the tip of the penis may be a tiny bit puffy or pink. It should not be swollen or *angry* red- this suggests a true infection of the foreskin called balanitis, that is much more common in uncircumcised boys. There may also be some drainage of pus. Balanitis requires antibiotics, as does a true urine infection. These conditions may also cause fever, abdominal pain and vomiting.

Your care provider can sort out a urine infection from irritation with a simple urine test. Once it is confirmed, irritation can be treated in boys with improved hygiene- shaking, that is- and a few days of some *Vaseline* applied to the tip of the penis. For girls, a bath with a cup of vinegar daily is an excellent natural healer. For both boys and girls, it may be necessary to retrain the bladder (or more correctly, the brain), so that they stop going potty every five minutes. This can be done by setting a timer for 10 minutes, then 15 etc.

Wetness can cause another problem in little girls. When the left and right sides of the labia are in constant contact, the cycle of wetness followed by drying can lead to the two sides sticking together. This is called labial adhesions. I think of this like a book that is left out in the rain- when the pages dry, they will stick together. Similarly, when the labia are in complete contact, then become wet followed by dry, they will also stick together. This sticking together will narrow the opening of the vagina. The reduction in the opening can be minor or almost complete. When it is severe, urine can pool behind the adhesions in the vagina. Occasionally urinary infection will result.

I am not aware of any scientific study of the prevention of labial adhesions, but I do have a theory. Many parents these days are taught not to clean between the labia when doing diaper changes because it is "self-cleaning". This is generally true, but if the labia are never separated, it makes sense that they would be more prone to sticking. I recommend that a washcloth be gently wiped between the labia every few days. Using a washcloth will avoid any irritants in baby wipes.

Once adhesions develop, there are different views on how they should be handled. Most doctors agree that if there is a severe narrowing of the labia, and if urinary infection has resulted, that active treatment should be started. The doctor can prescribe a vaginal cream that contains estrogen. Over days to weeks, the estrogen will soften the labia such that the adhesions break and the labia separate. Some doctors also recommend this treatment for less severe adhesions. Others, including myself, do not fret too much over mild adhesions. Rather than using medication, I recommend a small smear of *Vaseline* placed between the labia once a day while changing the diaper. You can then gently stretch the outer labia apart. Force should never be applied, as forcibly separating the adhesions is painful. The worst-case scenario has to start estrogen late. The adhesions will certainly resolve when her own estrogen kicks in.

And now, if you'll excuse me, I have to go pee.

Chapter 5: Everyone blooms

a.   It's amazing that development is as consistent as it is.

Think about it. Each year, about 135 million babies are born worldwide (1). One hundred and thirty-five million unique individuals each with his or her own identity. And yet, kids across the world follow more or less the same stages in their development. How cool is that? How boring would the world be if we all ended up exactly the same? It is by taking different paths that we learn unique skills and bring unique experience. In order for our individual traits to come out as we grow, we must take our own developmental path.

Each step in a baby's development brings her a little further on her journey in life. As adults, we talk a lot about a baby's milestones-sitting, crawling, walking etc. – because these are easy for us to track. I like to think about it much more as a progression. For example, tummy time allows her to lift her head and arms up. When the arms get strong enough, she pushes and rolls over. Strong arms allow the legs to start their work, and before you know it she is up on all fours. After a couple of months of spinning her wheels, she is crawling, and then pulling to stand, then cruising, and then walking. Before you know it, you are chasing her around the house.

We can go through the same sort of progression for using the hands, for language, and for socialization, although the time course is different. While most of us think about this process for just the first few years, it really continues on throughout childhood, and even into adulthood if we are continuing to learn. Each one of us will go to different lengths along a specific developmental pathway. We may become specialized in the coordination that it takes to skate or dance. We might develop the fine motor skills of a pianist or a surgeon. It depends upon our opportunities, our interests and the help of more experienced people around us.

We are the coaches and instructors for our kids. We give the opportunity to practice tummy time and other skills. However, since she does not read development or parenting books; she may not progress exactly the way the experts say. For example, if mobility is her goal, most will crawl first. Some will do it commando style. Some get right up on hands and feet, without touching their knees or elbows. Others roll or scoot on their bums. All of these methods meet the goal of mobility. Eventually we all get to walking and running because it is more efficient, but kids are not always too worried about that at first.

Some of the traits will be genetic. A few years ago, I met a two-year-old whose parents were concerned about his lack of speech. After spending time with them, it seemed very likely that he was a normal boy who just didn't talk very much. Near the end of the visit, it dawned on me that his father had barely said a word in thirty minutes. Sometimes apples fall close to trees, and when I expressed this thought, his parents chuckled with relief.

As an aside, it is important to talk to your children. This is an example of how the environment can affect a baby's development. Babies can actually detect the difference between their parent(s)' language and another spoken language before 4 days of age (1). Young children to whom parents speak more frequently will do better developmentally. If a baby is spoken to in more than one language, she will learn both the languages best as a young child. Interestingly, the first words for both languages may come a little later, just because she is processing two languages at once. She will quickly catch up in both and then have a tremendous gift to last a lifetime.

The pediatrician's job is to know when a child is far enough off the developmental path that concern should be raised. Just as with medical illnesses, it is better to err on the side of caution. It is usually better to pursue a delay in development than it is to wait too long. We know that early treatment for developmental issues leads to better outcomes. Experienced providers become comfortable with some of the less common, but still normal, patterns of development. Still, there is always that child who manages to do something unique.

So, should you stress your child is the last one in the playgroup to talk or walk? Probably not, even though most of us do. Remember, life is truly not a race. Development is the sum of multiple skills, not each skill in isolation. Besides, it is not always best to be early. An eight-month-old walker is like a drunk driver- all of the mobility, but none of the judgment.

b.   Baby Talk is not always talk

In the old cartoon, *The Magic School Bus*, the characters become tiny and are able to travel all over the body. Personally, if given this ability, I would go into a baby's brain. It would be a remarkable adventure. What marvels of activity and growth would await? How great would it be to learn the ways they think and communicate?

In the meantime, we will have to rely on what neuroscientists tell us. I use the word communicate, rather than *talk*, because babies don't use words. According to Dr. Kevin Nugent, a psychologist at the Brazelton Institute in Boston, we can understand how newborns communicate, if we observe them closely.

Some of what babies say is vocal, if not verbal. Crying is the most obvious form of baby talk. Babies cry to tell us when something makes them unhappy. As we discussed, an attentive parent will often learn the difference between the hungry cry, the tired cry and the pain cry. Some babies also have an angry cry that sounds more

135

like a cat's snarl. Conversely, they laugh. This comes a little later, usually at about 2 months of age. Laughing babies communicate joy to all around them. Not all babies laugh a lot, though the same as with adults. In between the extremes of laughing and crying, there is the *coo*, which is a lovely musical sound that has an early speech quality.

If you are patient, and your baby is quiet but alert, you might be able to engage him in conversation, even at an early age. Look him right in the eye and say, "Hello, baby. How are you?" in a cheerful voice. Then just stare, smile and wait. Your first reply will probably take close to a minute, and will be in the form of a brief coo. It is almost as if he is looking for the speech button in his brain, and being that it is new, it takes a while for him to find. Once he has answered, you speak briefly again. The second reply will probably be a little quicker, and soon enough a full-blown conversation will begin. Keep eye contact and a smile throughout this time. You will have no idea what he is saying, except that it is really good and important to him. Everyone should be so lucky as to hear a happy cooing baby.

It is important to listen to a baby with your eyes. This is where most of the communication can be found. If I put my cold hand on a newborn baby, he will shudder. If I undress him or try to straighten his legs, he will fidget. If I hold him in an awkward way, he will arch, and if I make him more comfortable, you can see (and feel) the tension disappear from his body. These are all ways of

136

expressing his likes and dislikes. As parents, you can listen to these cues so often that you become experts at understanding him. When spoon-feeding begins, you may find him open his mouth and lean towards you like a baby bird, or you may find he turns away and spits out what you have offered. He will speak in similar ways during other parts of his day.

There are many books and websites to describe exactly which sounds a baby will make at what age. I encourage you to also focus on the big picture, not just specific *sounds* but *communication*. If you have an eighteen-month-old that speaks a language that I call *toddler*, he may well sound almost completely garbled. For example, "Frabaga bra bugghaga daba truck" clearly is a full sentence about trucks, just not in English. I maintain that babies are smarter than adults. Since we cannot learn his language, in time, he learns ours. You do not have to rush the process- eat it up while it lasts. I can assure you that swearing in *toddler* can be just as explicit as it is in other languages- we hear it often when giving shots.

With time, he will gradually convert over to our language. The pace will vary depending on many things. Read and speak to him a lot. Teach him a second language right away if you know it. If he understands instructions well, hears well and is social, don't sweat too much if the words are slow to come. If understanding, hearing or socializing is an issue, follow-up early.

When *lellow* comes out for yellow, enjoy it while it lasts. And listen with your eyes, too.

c. If the doctor says your child is autistic, she probably is

Autism is a really difficult problem for a child to have and for a family to manage. Although there is a whole range of severities, the common elements are difficulties with language, socialization, and anxiety. Some children have severe speech delays and have difficulty making any words that can be understood. Others are very intelligent, but have trouble using language socially. A child might even name her letters early, but have no idea how to use letters to make language. Some children have fascinations with certain objects, and some have special skills in isolated areas, such as memory.

We know that autism is becoming more common, and about 1 in 150 children are affected. We do not know why this is the case. There are likely many reasons for the increase, including better awareness, and differences in how doctors use the term now, compared to in the past. There are clearly also other reasons that we do not understand. One thing is certain; when it is your child who is diagnosed, the numbers do not matter.

There is no cure for autism; it is a life-long condition. However, we know that early diagnosis and developmental intervention can really help improve a person's ability to function. Early diagnosis to me means during the second year. It is very difficult to detect in the first year. Some insightful parents of autistic children will look back and recognize behaviors such as poor eye contact, extreme anxiety around strangers, or being content while staring at a mobile for hours. Usually, the diagnosis is made when there is a delay in language skills and a lack of normal social skills. Some of these children will be less interested in what is going on around them. Many times parents will come to health care providers with these concerns. Other times, as providers, we will notice behaviors that give us concerns.

As a doctor, diagnosing autism often relies on a *sixth sense*. There are times during a child's visit when something just tells me that there is a problem. It can be difficult to put this sense into words. One of the clues is extreme anxiety about the doctor or doctor's office, keeping in mind that most toddlers hate the place where they get shots. There have been times when I literally could not get an autistic child in the examination room, and had to do the visit in the hallway. Other times, the child may have hand flapping, or speech which parrots what we just said. Instead of speaking, he may make musical sounds.

Whenever possible, I like to allow parents time to get their heads around a non-urgent diagnosis. For effective treatment of a condition, the patient (or parent) needs to *buy in* and agree with a caregiver's recommendations. Development delays, in general, and autism, in particular, do not give me this luxury. I have thought many times that the *second* worst thing I could do is to tell an unsuspecting mother and father that their child is autistic. The only thing worse would be to not tell them of my suspicions, because this will delay treatment, and delayed treatment denies a child his best opportunity for success.

This conversation can go very badly. It certainly can create a large rift between a family and me. Some people will choose to go see another provider, which is very understandable. At times, a doctor has to be the bad cop for the benefit of the child. One advantage of aging is to have a chance to see some of these children years later, and to have a parent thank me for the push towards treatment.

Doctors and parents are not the only ones who can be on different pages. A relative with experience caring for children may have insight prior to a parent, and may have to be the one who raises the subject. This is exceptionally hard, as it is for a preschool teacher or daycare provider. And perhaps worst of all is when spouses do not agree about a problem. Relationships are put under tremendous strain when one parent refuses to seek help that the other parent feels certain is needed. Separation and divorce can result. It is such a difficult time.

There is no good way to handle serious medical diagnoses, but having your eyes wide open is usually helpful. There will be a period of grief that follows this sort of news. You need to have permission to feel this grief, but at the same time, you need to help your child as early as possible. A good primary care provider can be your ally, by supporting you, and connecting you with services that will lead to the best possible outcome.

d. Treat learning disabilities early

A four-year-old boy comes in for his well visit. His mother says he is very bright but is not learning his letters the way that his sister did. The mother, who is also bright, wonders if he might have dyslexia. This is a very challenging question to answer. A four-year-old is not expected to know all his letters. Still, in this case, it seemed worth pursuing. Within a year, he is diagnosed with a learning disorder. He learns to read with a special technique, and never goes through the frustration of being left behind by his classmates. Today he is doing well as a high school senior.

Contrast this to another encounter. An eighteen-year-old is struggling to complete high school. He has a C average in general level classes, but it turns out he cannot read. He listens to books on tape to try to keep up. Testing reveals that he has a 160 IQ (genius level), but severe dyslexia. He had slipped through the cracks because he sat in the back and never complained.

Somewhere in between these two extremes are most kids with learning disorders. Most fall behind in the early years of school, and then get some testing. Most are labeled with a form of learning disability, some more precisely than others. Through extra help and tutoring, they are able to do reasonably well in school, but this is highly variable.

I do not want to suggest that every four-year-old who has yet to learn his letters needs to see a specialist, nor to imply that there is anything wrong with C's in general level courses. In fact, C's are average, and average describes most of us. (grading in school is a whole other issue that we could discuss for days.) The take-home message is that if you notice that one or more academic skill lags far behind your child's overall abilities, there may be a concern for a learning disability.

We should clarify some definitions. *Intelligence* is your overall thinking ability or potential. Consider it like the whole brain. People with high intelligence are smart; people with low intelligence have overall problems with thinking and learning. A *learning disability (or disorder)* is a specific problem with one or a few specific areas of learning. We group them by the particular difficulties experienced by the child. We talk about these being language-based (reading/writing or both) or math-based. These are particular short-circuits in an otherwise high functioning brain. *Dyslexia* is a language-based disability; most people think of it as reversing letters, but this term is often used interchangeably with any leaning disability of language.

IQ tests in people with learning disabilities will often have scores in one area which are considerably lower than all the others. In the next 50 years, our understanding of genetics and the brain will greatly increase. When this happens, we will have much more specific ways to categorize, diagnose and treat learning disabilities.

You do not need to worry about any of this. That is for neuroscientists. Instead, you can focus on reading to your children every day. See what skills they are learning. Report them to your provider at well visits. Listen to feedback from preschool teachers, as well as from people in your family who are experienced with children. If red flags are raised to these people, have an assessment done. There is nothing to lose.

If this seems overwhelming, I don't blame you. We have been talking this entire book about how wide is the range of normal development, the differences between boys and girls, and also how too much advice can be confusing. This is a hard area for a layperson to trust their gut. Even for child specialists- teachers, psychologists and doctors, learning disabilities are difficult to understand.

The best advice I can give is to be on the lookout, especially if disabilities run in the family. If there is an issue, it will clarify itself soon enough to make a big difference.

e. Teach your child a skill that makes her stand out

We all want our children to succeed in life. Success can be defined in many ways, and my most basic definition of successful is simply this: happy and safe. One of the keys to happiness is to be fulfilled, and it would be nice for your child to do something she considers to be meaningful and fulfilling. Although society tends to drive us to fit in, to be like others, and to do what others do, it is often a unique skill that sets us apart in the adult world, and makes us special. In some ways, the best time to begin to learn a skill is in infancy.

I am going to take a brief detour to talk about brain development, so that this discussion makes a little more sense. In the early weeks and months of life, the brain is growing quickly. Think about this- the head reaches 90 percent of its adult size by age 2! After this burst of growth of brain cells, the next process is referred to as pruning. Just like a gardener will prune a shrub, the brain will prune nerve connections that are unused, and reinforces ones that are used.

Have you ever tried to learn a second language as an adult? It usually does not come easy. Even in middle school, learning to roll a Spanish 'r' can be a constant challenge. On the other hand, young children who grow up in bilingual homes will speak both equally well. This difference occurs because young children have the potential to speak any language, but over time our ability to make certain sounds decreases if we have not been hearing them regularly. So, if your home is bilingual, the ideal time to teach your child both languages is right from birth. Ideally, if one of you speaks to her in one language, and the other in another language, it makes it easier for her to sort out which goes with which. If you are both unilingual, and a grandparent, friend or neighbor speaks a different language, by all means invite them to speak to your baby.

Perhaps you live near a ski hill, an ice arena or a golf course. Why not start them early? Small kids don't have far to fall and if they are supervised appropriately, can take part very safely. Just make sure you stretch your back, because bending over to help them takes its toll. If sports are not your thing, maybe music is instead.

My community has many scientists, due to the presence of the Woods Hole Oceanographic Institution. Currently, my patients include a three-year-old who has built eight robots with his father. He recently told me that " the motherboard is the brains of the computer" (clearly, he has a big motherboard, too.) The point is that if we teach our children what we know and love, we can provide them with both quality time and a special skill, at an age when the brain is specially equipped to learn.

I need to be clear that pressuring a child is not a good idea. We are not trying to create the next Mozart or Tiger Woods. I would not recommend an activity that a child clearly dislikes, activities that involve flash cards or their computer counterparts, nor sitting in a classroom at age 2 for Mandarin lessons. The difference between this and my young computer wizard is that the learning occurs in an environment where play comes first. Because his father loves computer gadgets, he can share his love while teaching his son. In other words, it has to be fun first.

The take home message is that the early years provide a unique opportunity to teach our children skills that can help them and provide enjoyment over a lifetime. If you teach them carefully, they will be grateful.

f.   Infants come from planets, too

A mildly distraught mother of a three-year-old boy recently came in for a well visit. "He always wants to wrestle with me", she said.
 "Is he angry or playing?", I asked. When she replied that he was playing, I suspected that the mother had not grown up with brothers. "What do the men in his life think of him?" was my next question.

"His uncle thinks he is awesome", was the reply. This was a Mars moment.

Some girls are Venetian. Some boys are definitely Martians. Some are in between on Earth, and a few swap planets. Every child is entitled to, and may normally act like he is from any planet. It is just that certain behaviors are much more common in boys and others are more common in girls. This is no less true than saying premature baby males are more likely to develop breathing problems, or teenage girls are more likely to develop rheumatoid arthritis. Admitting this helps us to better understand how children act.

How much of our behavior is genetic and how much is learned? Sociologists and psychologists have debated *nature versus nurture* for years. Both are undoubtedly important, and I have no desire to dive into this subject in great detail. A couple of common sense thoughts seem to suffice. First, we are born with certain personality traits. Think of this as the planet from which we come. Then, the influence of our environment- that is, our parents, families, caregivers and everything around us, pushes us to one part of the planet or another. This modifies our traits and leads to our final personalities. Our environment can push us to a certain extent, but it cannot push a Jupiter person to Saturn or vice versa.

The younger we are, the less time our environment has had to work on us. Babies are like clay- they start off a certain shape and soak up their exposures. They have primitive materials, which have yet to be molded into a final shape. In some ways, we may not be able to tell how they will turn out. In other ways, you see them as they truly are, without being covered by veneers. They do not cover their feelings, or act a certain way because of a sense of obligation or for some secondary gain. What you see is what you get.

I have seen eighteen-month-old girls nurse their dolls while their mothers nurse a younger sibling. I have seen several six-month-old boys examine my flashlight in three dimensions, as if they were not just fascinated by the light, but trying to figure out how it worked. In twenty years, I have not seen this from a girl. Surely, some of you out there have, and perhaps my observations are biased by prejudices, but it has not been for a lack of looking. Seeing these behaviors is equally fascinating both for its gender preference, and for the early age at which a sophisticated behavior seems to be occurring.

There is absolutely no need to worry if your child's behavior is not stereotypical, any more than there is need to worry if it is. I have been known to say that there are four basic types of boys- ball boys, truck boys, ball and truck boys, and those that like neither balls nor trucks. Some people call the ball and truck boys *all boy*; rather than being a value judgment, it is just a statement. Similar statements can be said of girls. We are all familiar with girly girls, as well as tomboys, including the baby sister with several older

148

brothers, who can beat the living daylights out of all of them. These days, we should probably add a computer boy and girl group. In reality, there is a much bigger spectrum of behaviors than a few groups can accurately depict, but categories do make it easier for us to understand personality types, as long as we don't put restrictions or expectations on the kids.

One last example that stands out. Two very concerned parents had perplexed expressions as they came in to their twin eighteen-month-olds well visits. The had gone to great lengths to raise their children gender neutrally -offering both the girl and the boy trucks and dolls, books and balls. To their amazement, the girl could already say, "Me go *Wal-Mart*", and she liked it there. The boy, in contrast, said only a few words like "Woof", "Vroom, vroom", "Mama" and "Dada". He did not like *Wal-Mart*, but he did like *Home Depot!*

You can't make stuff like that up.

Chapter 6: Good as gold

a. Weaning night feedings- the baby's first gift to his family

If someone made me a steak and cheese sandwich every night at 1 am, I would wake up and eat it. Throw in a chocolate milkshake and I'd make room for that, too. If, after six straight months of feeding bliss, that late night snack was suddenly taken away, I would almost certainly complain for a day or two. However, that doesn't mean I really needed it.

The situation for an infant is not so different. Of course, in the early weeks and months, nighttime feeding can be an essential part of a baby's nutrition. A newborn is encouraged to feed at least every three hours. We want to make sure that he can gain weight well. This is especially true when breastfeeding, when frequent feeding helps to stimulate the breast to produce milk. Babies with special nutritional concerns, like those who are premature or are small, may need to continue this pattern. Most are gradually able to stretch out the time between feedings in the first few months.

Advice on sleep is something that pediatricians can do in their sleep. And yet, it is still one of the most difficult subjects we discuss. Let's face it, sleep is important. Recommendations from experts about how we nurture our babies have changed, from tough love and crying it out, all the way to *baby whispering*.

Changes in expert opinion reflect inconsistencies in what doctors recommend to parents and society, only to have experts change opinions and approaches and…..

I went back and reviewed recent research on getting babies to sleep. A few things stood out. The first and most clear is that a baby should not co-sleep with parents. Co-sleeping almost triples the risk of Sudden Infant Death Syndrome (SIDS) (1). Next, there is some evidence to suggest that holding, feeding and rocking a baby to sleep in early infancy may lead to an increased likelihood of waking in later infancy. In contrast, routines at bedtime and attempts to put a baby down awake may lessen later waking issues. In addition, a *top up* feed between 10 pm and midnight may also allow babies to sleep longer afterwards. Finally, *crying it out* is also a successful method for reducing nighttime waking (2).

Every baby is his own person and will feed on his own timetable, unless one is imposed on him. Many parents tolerate frequent daytime feedings if the baby is sleeping fairly well at night. Allowing the baby to dictate the schedule and get to sleeping through the night on his own time is what I call *the low road*. It avoids confrontation. Unfortunately, not all babies want to take this road. Some young babies just did not read this chapter of the book. No matter how careful you are as a parent, he may fall asleep during the last feed of the day. Or he might not go to sleep until you rock him. Almost everyone would agree that this is appropriate in the first few months. If it persists, you may need to take *the high road*, by letting them cry it out. Most mothers do not at all want to have their babies endure prolonged crying. As a rule of thumb, I don't bring up the subject of crying it out until at least six months.

Occasionally, a parent cannot wait that long. By 4 months, it is certainly reasonable to only feed the baby once at night. Keep in mind that not everyone has the same definition of a night. I call it a period of at least eight hours, whether that is 11 pm to 7 am or 8 pm to 4 pm. In other words, by 4 months, it is reasonable to expect healthy babies to go at least four hours without feeding. To be honest, most can go six hours. Eight is pushing it for some. The trouble with trying to wean a baby to only one night feed is that it is just as difficult as weaning them to zero feeds. It always seems to me a little unreasonable for us to say, "If you wake *this once* in the night, you can be fed, but if you wake *twice*, you're out of luck." For this reason, most parents wait until the baby is a little older, and get the whole night solved, if necessary.

I often joke with parents that you are ready to let the baby cry if your fatigue level is higher than the baby's need for nighttime nutrition (any time after 6 months). However you do it, the baby will probably protest at first. It is really important to be ready for the change because it is not easy. *Be prepared for 60 to 90 minutes of crying three nights in a row.* Night 1 is usually bad, but night 2 is worse because the baby is exhausted and determined at the same time. It is amazing that by night 3, the vast majority of babies will get there. If you are not ready for three nights, it is best to wait, since you will get all of the pain and none of the gain. The same goes if you object on principle. It is a long time to listen to your baby cry. It is perfectly reasonable to not want to do it this way. You then just go back to the low road.

Many people are familiar with the method where the parent briefly goes back in the room after five minutes, then 10 minutes, then 15 etc. I don't usually recommend this because a baby that is just about to settle can be re-energized by the sight of his parent. If you feel the need to listen in, put a monitor in the room and suffer from a distance.

If you go the cry it out route, a few important tidbits that can help make the transition smoother. First, plan ahead. Choosing a time when there is no company, no job interviews or major holidays increases the chances of success. Let the neighbors know, if you live in an apartment. Second, there are some super stubborn babies that just refuse to give in. I usually set an upper limit of two hours of crying, and thankfully that probably happens much less than one percent of the time. Third, be aware of a few things that baby may do to up the ante. Some babies cry to the point of throwing up. If this happens, you are not mean if you clean up the baby and the crib, give a quick kiss, and start again. I sometimes advise people to have a crib sheet, change of clothes and diaper ready if they suspect this will happen. One step worse is the baby that bangs his head from being upset. The champion at inducing parental guilt is the guy who cries to the point of holding his breath and passing out. Yes, that really happens, but fortunately it is harmless and does not occur very often. Unfortunately, some really smart babies will learn to manipulate these strategies.

It is common for a setback to occur some weeks after you achieve success, similar to an adult who has quit smoking. For babies, it is usually triggered by teething, an ear infection, or some other illness. It may require starting from scratch with crying it out, but most of the time it is much quicker to achieve success the second time around. You may find that he starts off sick, and finishes off just wanting to be held at night. You can tell that the cry is for attention if it stops the moment the baby is picked up. If a baby is in pain, he will probably fuss for much longer, or until something is done to relieve the pain.

Finally, some parents worry that their child will be emotionally scarred by having to cry for an extended period of time. I do not worry about this. You might think this is a hypocritical recommendation from the same person that says you will not spoil a baby by holding him. From my perspective, by giving comfort and affection ninety nine percent of the time, your baby will learn that he is loved and he can trust. He is the center of the universe. Even if learning to sleep at night means tough love, he is acknowledging that there are a few other stars out there too, and among them are Mom and Dad. Don't forget that we are all better parents with a better night's sleep. And I really think that the only way he will learn to overcome the feeling that the *sun is never going to come up again,* is to feel that the sun is never going to come up again. But sure enough, it does. When morning comes, you are there to greet, comfort and congratulate him on his sleep, and his resilience. Rest assured.

b. Toddler and preschooler sleep problems- the loaf of bread technique

"I'm scared."

" I have to go to the bathroom."

"I heard a noise-did you hear that? "

"I need to tell you something." "What?" " Um, um, um…. I forget."

I remember hearing that age 4 is the most common time for children to have trouble going down to sleep and staying in bed for the night. This makes sense in light of the explosion of imagination that takes places in a child's mind at that age. It also coincides with a huge growth of new nerve cells in the toddler/preschooler brain. To be honest, though, it seems like every age can be challenging for some children to sleep well. In the next few paragraphs, I am going to review a technique that works well for young children, essentially 18 months to 4 years. No surprise that this is the same age when they learn (and perfect) climbing out of the crib or bed.

A good bedtime routine goes a long way. It helps to prepare your child for her bedtime. It can be a great family time in an otherwise busy life. It usually involves some combination of bath, teeth, stories and cuddling, but certainly can include other activities that your family likes- singing song, for example. For a parent, the bedtime routine helps to wind down the child's day, and it also gives you a sense of wellbeing. This can also help you feel like less of a heel when you need to practice tough love.

Once it is time to go to sleep, you may want to have some snuggle time. This you will definitely miss once the children are older. If she is still in a crib, snuggling can be done in a chair. It is usually best to leave the room before she goes to sleep, so that she can learn to fall asleep on her own. Falling asleep on your own at bedtime helps her fall back asleep when she wakes up in the middle of the night.

When the waking up starts, and you find her in your room or at the top of the stairs, the challenge begins. The first decision is whether or not you will try to gate her in. If she is in a crib, there are *crib domes* that can be secured over the crib to prevent climbing out. Although I have been a fan of them in the past, recently concerns have been raised about whether the domes themselves pose a safety risk. Unfortunately, good studies are lacking. If she is in a bed, you may be able to get away with a gate on the door. Sometimes safety issues force you to use these physical barriers-for example, if you live in an old house with very steep or uneven stairs. Keep in mind, though, that necessity is the mother of invention, and kids will show their true ingenuity in the ways they break out of prison. I have often said that the only barrier that really can be trusted is the one inside the brain- hence, the *loaf of bread technique.*

It goes something like this. If you were to wake up one night and find a loaf of bread in your bed, it might seem a little odd. Even so, most of us would simply pick up the bread and return it to where it belongs in the kitchen. We would not feel sorry for it nor stress about the effect that sleeping in the kitchen would have on the bread's emotional development. If, a short time later, we were to once again find the bread in our bed, we would do the same thing. We would not yell at the bread. We would not say, "Loaf of bread, you are getting big now and you need to sleep in the kitchen." We would not cuddle it; we would simply hold it unemotionally, and return it to the kitchen. If this occurred 50 times, we would do the same.

The same basic technique works for children. With your child, you may want to preview the change in policy earlier in the day. Something like, "Starting tonight I want you to sleep in your own bed and I am not going to let you sleep with me." When bedtime comes, a quick reinforcement is a good idea (although it will not prevent most children from trying their usual tricks). When she does get up and ends up in your room, there may well be a litany of excuses about teeth, the bathroom, thirst, etc. Filling one of her requests is more than reasonable on your part. After that, the bread approach begins. Don't talk, yell, cuddle or otherwise get sucked in. Just put her back in bed. Repeat as many times as she reappears until you win. This could be 50 times.

By winning the first night, you have set a precedent. Subsequent nights become easier. You have created a barrier *inside her brain*, so that she now believes it is not worth the effort of repeated trips into Mommy and/or Daddy's room. When she does go a whole night without a visit to you, be sure to praise her, and give a sticker or some other reinforcement. After a week or two of stickers, some reward (which does not involve being in your room) is helpful.

Remember, we are all better parents with a good night's sleep. And even though the baker is an early riser, she still doesn't sleep with the loaves of bread.

c. Toddlers are only 3000 tantrums away from a more functional behavior

As you can tell, I like to joke around a lot with parents. It is my way of saying that everything is OK, or will be OK, no matter how it seems at the moment. So when I say the line about the 3000 tantrums, a lot of parents of toddlers look at me as if to say, "Yeah,

158

that's not really funny", and I reply, "I wasn't actually joking about this one."

Tantrums are classically thought of as part of the terrible twos. Occasionally, they start in infancy- these are the truly feisty babies. Some fifteen-month-olds have full on temper tantrums. I tell these parents that their children are *advanced*, in the same way as if they talk or walk early. After all, there has to be something positive about it. It is not unusual to see these kids move out of the tantrum stage earlier, too. I will never forget that my otherwise happy youngest son, Christopher, woke up on his second birthday and had two tantrums before breakfast. We joked that his biological clock was working.

Some kids are delightful as two-year-olds, only to become beasts at 3. Three and 4 are like *2 on steroids* for some kids. The tantrums are more intense and the talk which accompanies the tantrums is much more descriptive. The parents of these kids need a headphone and earplug, which translates, like the ones at the United Nations. That way, when he says, "I hate you", you can translate to, "Mommy, you were right, I should have gone to sleep when you told me, and yes, I am a complete grouch when I don't eat my breakfast." No wonder that one father in my practice told me, "The terrible twos are nothing compared to the f******* threes!"

At whichever age you are experiencing this joy, take consolation in the fact that it will pass if handled well. Surviving tantrums involves what I like to call the four C's. The first C is consistency-if your child knows the rules, then he at least has a chance to follow them. It is OK that he does not follow them regularly, because this process usually takes months to years rather than days to weeks. One of the most important components of consistency is that you will not give in to tantrums. This is akin to negotiating with terrorists. In fact, the best thing you can do is to leave the room (provided it is safe to do so). If he seeks you out and acts out further with hitting or other bad behavior, you may have to up the ante with a time out (see next chapter). Otherwise, tantrums are best left alone. Eventually, he will realize the behavior is not working and move on. If you are tempted to try and talk him through it, ask yourself how that would have worked for you the last time you were absolutely furious.

The second C is compassion. They aren't being obnoxious on purpose, and remembering this helps. Except when they are being obnoxious on purpose, at which time it is the parents right to bust them, figuratively speaking.

The third C is common sense. If you try to take your two-year-old to Wal-Mart at 5 pm, do not expect it to end well. Sometimes you still have to, but be ready for the consequences.

The final C is *Calgon*. With apologies to those too young to remember the ad with the mother who escapes to her bubble bath, we all need a chance to decompress. It may be putting ourselves in

160

time-out, going to the gym, an occasional date night, or night out with guys or girls. It could even be sitting in the car with the windows up and crying or yelling for five minutes. As long as it is not destructive, a little break can go a long way.

You will look back one day at this period and laugh, but you might not when you are in the middle of it. And remember, if you are tempted to give in to tantrums, think about how it would look to see him having them at fourteen. This should give you the will to stay strong.

d. Time Out: for works in progress

Doctors and child psychiatrists will tell you that it is more helpful to reward good behavior than to punish bad behavior. Attention from you is very important to your child, and you want to show him that good behavior gets the most attention. This will encourage the good action to occur again.

That being said, all parents eventually face the struggle of how to discourage unwanted behaviors. One standard way is to divide these behaviors into three groups. The first group is behaviors that are best ignored. This includes tugging on your leg, attention seeking and tantrums. By ignoring these actions, they will usually become less common. Remember that it takes months, not days.

The other extreme is those infractions bad enough to warrant punishment without a warning or second chance. This is the truly obnoxious group, for things such as hitting, biting, spitting, swearing and other wonderful things that you never imagined your offspring could do. And yes, it is not just your child who does this! For these, I suggest a *time out with no warning* because it tells the child that he has done something big, not in a good way. In a sense, it creates a special category for violence and aggression.

The in-between group consists of behaviors bad enough to warrant discouragement, but for which a second or third chance should be given before punishment. It may be things such as throwing food or cups, or deliberately not listening. There are a couple of ways to handle these actions. For toddlers, you will mainly be redirecting them away from what they are doing. "No, no, leave the plug. No, No stay away from the stairs", and so on. You will sound like a broken record, but this repeated teaching is how he will learn. As he reaches 2 and older, redirection may gradually be replaced at times by warnings. If the warnings are not heeded, then the child may lose what he is playing with, or be put into *time out*.

Enforcing a time out can be done in several ways. I am a product of the old 1-2 3 Magic school, and will describe essentially that method (1). First, you need to choose a time out spot. It can be a chair, a step or even the child's room. I do not believe that you will scar your child by doing time out in his room. As long as most of his experiences in his room are positive, a time out or 200 will not hurt. Still, this is your choice. There is something to be said for picking a chair or a step, as these are easy to find when you are not at home.

When sending your child to time out, it doesn't matter if you say, "That's 1, that's 2, that's 3. You're in time out." After a while, I found that annoying, and just said, "No", the first time, "if you do that again you're going to time out", the second time, and "you need to go to time out", the third time. It seems like more normal conversation to me.

Regardless of which words you use, two things are important. The first is to limit your talking. Saying, " Mommy loves you and you need to be a nice boy and yada yada yada…" is providing too much attention for negative behavior. So is laughing or getting angry. Remember, the most underrated sign of intelligence is a child's ability to pull his parent's strings, and the second most underrated is the ability to get himself in trouble. Combining those two is the ultimate coup de gras for a child. As a result, a poker face and a minimum of talking are recommended. Even if you have to go in another room to cry, or in the car to scream at some point, do not show him how amused or angry you are. I realize how this can be extremely difficult.

Once in time out, many kids will not stay put at first. A similar approach works. Tell him first that he needs to stay in time out, next that if he doesn't stay put you are going to hold him, and finally, you hold him. On the way to picking him up, you can set a timer for the desired length of time (1 minute per year of age still works well.) Then put him in a bear hug and let the kicking and screaming begin. When the timer rings, briefly say, "You need to stop throwing the ball in the house", or whatever it was, and then quickly redirect him into a positive activity. Do not be surprised if you are hounded, get your leg tugged on, or are verbally challenged. Many kids will have a tantrum after this. Try to ignore it unless it involves hitting, biting or swearing, in which case you are back in time out.

The good news is that after a few episodes of this, the kicking and fighting will stop. A honeymoon period of sitting quietly in time out will likely follow, and then he will challenge you again by trying to get up out of his seat. Sometimes, you have to briefly redo the holding technique, but not for too long.

Time out is a great technique for young kids as long as it done exactly right. Consistency is really important. Sometimes I even suggest that you write out a small chart that has three lists of behaviors to *Ignore, Time Out with Warning,* and *Time Out No Warning.* That way, when it is 5 pm and the kids are screaming, you are making dinner and you are tired, you have it right there in front of you. It can also be useful to make sure couples are on the same page. This is especially true when there is split custody or daycare involved. Remember, too, that it is very easy to make one small mistake that seems to throw you off track. If this happens, just check in with your care provider; they can probably steer you back in a good direction without much effort. The full video or book version of 1,2,3 Magic is also worth the effort in these situations.

Finally, you have to be realistic about your goals. Time out will not single-handedly turn your child into an angel. I will always remember when we first used time out at my house. My middle child Andrew was 18 months old, and he started to hit Catherine, his three-year-old sister. Being a relatively new pediatrician, I confidently assured my wife that a solution was at hand. We started him in time out, and sure enough, within a week or two his behavior was changed. He had learned to hit his sister, and then sit himself down on the step for a minute thirty without being told! And being a nice older sister, she would go sit with him. The one silver lining was that when he started playing hockey, he knew exactly what to do when he got in trouble. Just go sit in the penalty box for a minute and a half.

e. Saying No allows them to appreciate Yes

I just finished Bobby Orr's remarkable new autobiography, appropriately titled Orr: My Story (1). In his own words, arguably the greatest hockey player ever, repeatedly discusses how fortunate he was, and how he is no better than anyone else. He gives the credit to those around him, especially his parents. And the main thing that his parents did for him was to treat him well, but not better than his siblings. When asked how her young son was doing, his mother, Arva, would say, "Which one? I have three." Take a minute to consider that- one of the great athletes of the last 100 years did not get special treatment at home. From years of living on Cape Cod, as he does, I have only ever heard kind words spoken of him. His parents raised a great person.

At heart, is that not what we all want for our children? Yet, somehow raising a good person often gets lost along the way. Parents almost always have good intentions, but many lose track of what really matters. I have seen parents at a kids' track meet step onto the track to photograph their kid, and block the track for another child. I have had a father furiously demand our last available flu shot for his perfectly healthy child, when it was saved for a child with a serious illness. I have seen parents whose son was nearly expelled, for threatening a school worker, lament, "I don't understand, we gave him everything." I have even seen people, who were waiting for a routine visit, complain because I was at the hospital caring for a child with life-threatening meningitis.

The link in all of these stories is the feeling of entitlement that develops when we never hear "No", and when we are allowed to feel that we are better than everyone else. Doctors are as guilty of acting entitled as any group of people, but those who are, learn this behavior as young children. I do not know exactly why our society has become more about *me* and less about *us*, but it is clear that there has been a distinct shift in this direction in the last 50 years.

I believe that the solution begins at home, and it begins in early childhood. As we have already discussed, the first year is the time when the baby gets almost everything she wants and needs. By about the age of nine months, the word "No" appears more often in our speech. This is usually when children start to move about the house and explore, getting into mischief and danger along the way. "No, no, no, leave the plug", and "No, no, no that's hot" are common examples. For parents, this is also a time when you feel like you are never sitting, because you essentially are never sitting. You follow your baby around the house like a spotter at the circus, keeping her safe.

By the second year, you have to deal with some or all of getting her to sleep, weaning from the breast or bottle, and weaning from a pacifier. These are what I call the *quit smoking goals of toddlerhood*, because they are about as difficult for the baby as quitting smoking is for an adult. Hopefully, the sleep issue has been handled months earlier, but this is often not the case. Typically, we have parents try to check them off one at a time, with a break of days to a couple of weeks in between for everyone to regroup. Just as with quitting smoking, it can be proceeding well, only to get side-tracked at a time of stress, like teething for sleep, or the stomach bug for the bottle. Most of the time, there will be a period of considerable upset on the baby's part; in other words, lots of crying. With perseverance, the baby will adapt.

167

In the process, she has learned an extremely important lesson. I have said before that the only way to learn that the sun will come up again, is to experience the feeling that it never will, but see that it does. In other words, it is just as important that you teach your baby resilience, as it is to get her to sleep or wean. This does not mean that you have to be cruel or hard-nosed. This teaching can be done with great compassion. Although your child will not remember these rights of passage later on, on some level, it will help her get through the terrible twos, and not getting the candy bar at the grocery check-out line, and even not getting the new cell phone later on. You, on the other hand, will remember every difficult behavior milestone, and thinking back to previous difficult struggles that ended well will help you build success upon success.

You know you have arrived when your adolescent starts to say things like, "That's so not fair!" and "How come all the other kids get to go, but I don't?"

The other part of limit setting is the idea that the feelings of other people also matter. When your daughter sleeps at night, she is doing something to help her parents. When she has to share a toy, she is doing the same for another child. Some kids achieve these goals much more easily than others; her temperament will definitely play a role. However, all children can learn to be good members of a group. I have heard mothers of toddlers and preschoolers say things like, "I don't mind so much if she hits me, it is when she does it to other people that it is a problem." This misses the point. Part of the role of a family is to teach a child how to act in the world at large. We practice at home, and then bring that experience to school and other places. Most children find it harder to be nice to their family than they do to others. In fact, don't be surprised if you feel like the progress with good behavior at home seems painfully slow. You will know you are on the right path if your preschool aged child gets good behavior reviews from the babysitter, teacher and grandparents. That is the feedback that will help you to stick with the program.

We need to get back to teaching our children what is truly important. Core values such as respect for your fellow man and putting others before yourself will take your child far in the important parts of life. And apparently, it doesn't hurt performance on the sports field, either. Just ask Bobby Orr.

f.   About *Energizer Bunnies*

"He is in perpetual motion."
"She climbs on everything."
"He has no fear."
"She doesn't seem to need to sleep."

Most children become busy once they start to move. In fact, the first six months after mobility begins, roughly age 9 to 15 months, is probably the most underrated busy time of parenthood. They seem to never stay still, and so, you never stay still. Even finding a safe time to go to the bathroom can be a challenge. Any opportunity to explore is taken, and what seems dangerous to us is often just part of the adventure for them. As my brother puts it, "The only true childproofing is direct supervision", but even a glance in the other direction can result in an escape up a staircase, down a hallway or onto a table.

Thankfully, most kids outgrow this stage. By age 2, her increased speed and mobility will be compensated by improved balance. Although you will still need to constantly watch her, most of the time you will not have to be the *spotter at the circus*, with each arm on either side of him. By age 3, she will probably be able to play independently, and your main role will be to verbally steer her out of harm's way.

In a moment of pride, you might even find yourself quoting Dr. Suess:
"You have brains in your head.
You have feet in your shoes
You can steer yourself
Any direction you choose.
You're on your own. And you know what you know.
And YOU are the guy who'll decide where to go." (1)

Except when you don't. Because, sometimes, you won't. I'm sorry to say it, it's hard, but it's true. An Energizer Bunny can happen to you.

Some children just never seem to stop moving. When age 2 and 3 comes, instead of becoming a little safer, they just become a lot faster. One young friend of mine was riding a two-wheeler by his second birthday- no training wheels! By age 4, he was trying to jump it off a retaining wall. As a teenager, he is now an accomplished athlete, but he continues to make his mother gray with his risk-taking antics, and he has wound up in the emergency room on several occasions.

How can a parent survive a non-stop kid like this, and make sure that the kid survives, too? It is not easy, but it can be done. Safety is the first consideration. You have to keep them constantly in your sight. You can arrange your space at home to help you. For example, toddlers like this are the reason that playpens were invented. There is absolutely nothing wrong with using physical barriers to keep him out of harm. Sooner or later, and probably sooner, she will learn to climb out of this and out of the crib. When this happens, you may want to get a *crib dome*, but these sometimes have their own safety issues. While awake, you can try to have her in a safe room, which has been super childproofed, and from which she cannot escape, without going directly past you. These are kids whose parents put the kitchen chairs in the garage

171

or laying down flat on the floor, so that they cannot be used as ladders.

Escape artists are a particular concern. Windows need to have childproof locks. Balconies and decks must be inaccessible. Front doors may need some kind of security system. For those who cannot afford a professional system, a cowbell hung on the door can sound an alarm. If you live on a busy street, you have to make sure Houdini is kept out of the road.

Shopping can be a nightmare. Some parents resort to a harness and leash. Otherwise, it is not unusual for store displays to crash, for her to play hide and seek in the dress section while you panic, or for you to be chasing her down an aisle. Most go to great lengths to avoid bringing her at all. The problem is that very few baby-sitters will have the skills to watch her. This is not a job for a thirteen-year-old or an elderly grandparent.

In addition to physical barriers to escape, certain parenting styles can really make life easier. I like to call it the *nurturing drill sergeant.* You need to stay on top her, and redirect frequently, and provide structure for tasks. You will have to give one instruction at a time, and repeat it frequently. Try to think of her as having hearing trouble, rather than listening trouble. It is a lot easier to be forgiving if you think of it this way, and you are much less likely to get angry. Limit your number of rules as best you can, as this will make it easier to be consistent with the ones you have. And set up routines, so that there are plenty of chances for him to practice.

Preserving your sanity is also important. Get outside and play as often as possible. This will burn off some of his energy, and teach her a good outlet for later in life. Work as a couple to trade off and allow your partner to rest. If you are single, lean on energetic members of your family or take advantage of any community supports to which you have access. Enroll her in a preschool where the kids get outside a lot. A mother's helper can be invaluable to wear her out while you supervise and sit!

I have avoided the term hyperactive up to now, mainly because a high level of activity is normal at this age. However, there is a point when Attention Deficit Hyperactivity Disorder (ADHD) occasionally has to be considered. As an expert lecturer once explained, the only reasons to medicate a preschooler are if the child is going to jump out the window, the parent is going to jump out the window, or the parent is going to toss the child out the window.

If you're getting near that point, call your pediatrician.

g. Play

   With apologies to Shel Silverstein

There is an old activity
That's seldom seen of late.
You may not even know it
If you're less than twenty-eight.

It doesn't need a teacher,
A trainer or a coach.
These days it would be called
A non-traditional approach.

It may not help with Harvard,
Nor scouts from Major Leagues,
But do not underestimate
The ways it meets your needs.

It doesn't use computers,
A cursor or a mouse,
No need for new technology
You'll find around the house.

It might involve a butterfly,
A turtle or a puppy,
A kid can do it on his own
Or with a friend if lucky.

It doesn't have specific rules
Or if it does they vary,
Depending on if you're doing it
With Cole, Devaun or Kerry.

And most of all it can be done

Without grownups all around,
Without a big tuition
Or travel out of town.

Imagination is the key
To how this game is run.
What playing teaches kids the most
Is just how to have fun.

h.   You say, "Yes", they say, "No, no, no"

Children who object are perhaps the most challenging children to raise. There is something about defiance that seems personal. Known by terms such as strong-willed and obstinate, when at an extreme level, clinicians describe these kids as having Oppositional Defiant Disorder. They provoke an emotional response, which I am noticing even as I write this passage. In order to channel them in a positive direction, parents must overcome this emotion. It takes a special kind of parent and parenting style.

You will usually recognize his defiance emerging in the second year, although in retrospect you may recall that he had a temper even as an infant. He may seem inpatient, demanding and easily frustrated. This frustration can lead to hitting, biting and other physical aggression, especially if he is not yet able to use words. You may ask yourself what you are doing wrong, to which the answer is usually nothing at all.

My sense is that oppositional children are born, not made. According to the American Academy of Child and Adolescent Psychiatry (AACAP), "Most authorities believe that biological factors are important in ODD." (1) One stereotypical scenario is what I call the Ying-Yang couple- one parent who is very easy-going, and the other who is more demanding. Many times, there is no evidence at all of the tree from which the apple fell.

Remember that developing independence means having your own opinions. Saying *no* is an important ability for children to develop as they mature. This can be as normal as it is for a young child to be busy at the same age. However, just as most busy kids settle into preschool without becoming hyperactive, most can also emerge from the two's and three's without becoming angry all the time. Unfortunately, some children continue to struggle with this task.

How can you raise your oppositional child to be happy at home, and with his preschool peers? It is not easy, but it begins by recognizing that you are in a special parenting situation. If you are a novice with children, you are probably going to need help, whether it is from a health care provider, counselor, preschool teacher, or a family member who raised a similar child. There are several good books on the subject, which can be accessed through the AACAP (2). If your child not only objects, but repeatedly disintegrates into a long-lasting emotional state of chaos, The Explosive Child, by Ross Greene, PhD is an excellent choice (3).

The key to success is to defuse the anger through a combination of prevention, picking your battles and consistency. You will learn very quickly the importance a good routine that is not too busy. Surprises are not usually welcome by oppositional children. Missed sleep and missed meals will lead to disaster. You will always need to have a snack with you, in case of emergency (even though meltdowns rarely have anything to do with true low blood sugar).

It might seem easier in the short run to give in to his wishes, but as we all know, this will lead to a spoiled child who struggles in the adult world. Much more effective is to limit conflict by choosing your battles carefully. For example, safety issues are not negotiable. From there, it is a personal decision as to which behaviors you will deem unacceptable. Keeping the list reasonably short will make everyone's lives easier and happier.

Negotiation is a good technique for *middle of the road* conflicts. For example, when driving on the highway and he says, "I dropped my toy. You need to get it NOW!", you say, "I am not in a place where I can stop right now, but when we pull off the highway, I will get it for you." This will work a lot better than, "You do NOT talk to me like that." Similarly, when a meltdown is in full swing, parents learn that it may just be easier to bale on music class, than to force him in just because you already paid for the lesson. What you are trying to avoid are the days where you seem to go from one prolonged struggle to the next. These conflicts are extremely stressful. If you reach this point, it is time to seek professional help.

Helping these kids is a long, slow process. You will need good planning, wise decision-making, and a tremendous amount of patience. It is not unusual for one parent to be more patient than the other. Sometimes a good parent has to say, " You had better take over, because I am going to get angry." The less patient parent needs to try not to turf all of the responsibility, because this can lead to resentment in a couple, at a time when you need to be a team. You will also need breaks to decompress emotionally. Physical exercise can be a great outlet, as can help from close friends and family.

As difficult as this sounds, I am amazed by the skill, poise, grace and love with which many parents learn to handle their oppositional children. You and he will be eternally grateful that you took on the challenge.

i.   Drama begins in preschool

Maybe sooner.
And I would not believe it, if I had not seen it myself.

Webster's dictionary defines drama as "a state, situation, or series of events involving interesting or intense conflict of forces." (1)

When drama happens between people, it is certainly intense and conflicted. I definitely would not choose the word interesting, but there must be something at some level pleasurable that drives at least one of the parties to initiate it.

Some children are born with an amazing flare for the dramatic, shall we say. I have seen nine-month-olds scream bloody murder while I look in their ears, then stop immediately when I am done. Sometimes they even grin. Clearly, the crying was not pain; instead, the baby wanted to let me know that it was emotionally upsetting. Occasionally, I have suggested that a career on the stage might lurk on the horizon, and the parents usually laugh (although they might just be humoring me!)

Older kids involved in drama have been given names such as Bully, Queen Bee, Wannabee, Victim, Bystander and Hero. For young children, I think of each as being born with basic personality traits-mellow, high-strung, aggressive, anxious, happy, fussy- and the like. In the first years, these traits will be influenced by the way the child is treated by parents and other caregivers. We want all babies to be loved, held, spoken and sung to, and generally nurtured. This will bring out the best in them, whatever their traits may be.

In the second and third years, kids of a similar age generally begin to play with each other, whether they are at a home, in playgroups, or at daycare. The adults who watch them will quickly learn who is the aggressor in claiming toys, who hits or bites in retaliation, who cries, who does not leave the adult's side, and who plays alone, seemingly oblivious to the conflict unfolding nearby. All of these behaviors are normal at this age. Parents are often stressed to see their child as either aggressor or retaliator. Teaching cooperative social skills and simple problem solving is a great way to help the children. Sometimes the one who has the toy first gets to play with it, and sometimes it is the next person's turn. Sometimes it just better to have two of the same toy!

Parents can create completely unnecessary drama in these situations. An aggressor's parent may verbalize dismay, only to have another parent agree, when she should reassure. Or the aggressor's parent may not act to gently curtail the behavior, leaving the other parent in an awkward and potentially resentful position. Before you know it, a two-year-old has a *bad rep*! It is so much better if adults are honest and try to do the right thing. All children are going to have traits that need gentle bending; this is entirely normal. Parents need to be willing to work on social skills, without making excuses. Other parents need to refrain from blowing normal behaviors out of proportion.

Preschoolers gain an increasingly complex social repertoire. Interactions become more sophisticated. They move from playing in parallel with other kids to actively playing together. Imaginative and role-play emerges. As part of these roles, there are leaders and followers, and those who are assertive or shy. Conflicts will arise when kids have different ideas about how play should proceed.

Again, this offers many moments to teach cooperation and sharing. Children can now be given a framework or basic set of rules for how they should interact. For example, "You can play with the first toy you find until snack time. After snack, you have to find a different toy." Children begin to thrive on consistent rules at this age, and kindergarten becomes the ultimate time for rule following. I have always felt that every adult workplace should have a kindergartener, to explain the rules when adults cannot agree.

The more complex the interaction, the more opportunity for drama. Children can begin to become singled out, not only for how they act, but also in any way in which they differ from others. "Only kids with brown hair can sit at this station", would be an example. Primitive examples of bullies and the various other roles begin to emerge in a group. Adults play a key role in *peace-building*. Some children are natural peace-builders. Most others can easily be taught how to be inclusive, accepting, and cooperative. Praising the children for good social behavior is the best way to build upon it. Unfortunately, there will also be children who struggle. This may be due to the way the child is wired, because of the home environment, or both. About once a month, I have to deal with a child who has been kicked out of a preschool for poor behavior. Physical aggression is the number one offense which schools site. It just is not OK to hurt other children repeatedly. Some of these children will have Oppositional Defiant Disorder (see chapter 6h) and/or Attention Deficit Hyperactivity Disorder. Others will be witnesses to violence, or victims of neglect.

Most drama is emotional rather than physical. It does not lead to expulsion, just unhappiness. It can be much more subtle, as bullies can be sweet to many or even most other people, while being mean to a targeted child or children. The victims may be slow to come forward, and in the preschool age may show indirect symptoms such as anxiety, sadness or bellyaches. It is not unusual for bullying behavior to be learned from a parent, and it can be very frustrating for schools when the parent is unwilling to accept responsibility for his child's actions. Creative strategies may have to be used by the school to get buy-in. This can be a real test of the teacher's social skills. Fortunately, many preschool teachers are ninjas in this regard. After all, they are experts in behavior that resembles a developmental age of 4, even if it is coming from a parent!

Joking aside, it is important to understand that the seeds of bullying are planted early. We all know the unpleasant, and occasionally devastating, consequences that can ensue in the teen years when drama escalates. By gently teaching our children to be peace builders from an early age, and by modeling good behavior ourselves, we can keep the drama where it belongs- on the stage.

j.   When it comes to electronics, less is more

Electronic media pervade our entire lives. Some would say they *invade* our entire lives. Recent research suggests that even children under age 2 watch between one and two hours of television each day. Up to one in three three-year-olds has a television in his room. And children 8 and under spend almost four hours per day with a television on in their background (that is, with no one in particular watching it). The advent of smart phones and tablet computers makes it almost certain that that electronic media exposure will increase. For children, especially the young, there is a big potential downside to excessive media exposure. Many parents seem to be unaware of these risks. Pediatricians believe that this is a very important subject to discuss.

At an infant's check-up, I often parents ask if the baby likes books. This is a gentle way of asking about reading. Many times, the parents answer, "Oh yes, he loves them", but surprisingly often they say, "Oh, I haven't tried them yet. But he really likes the TV and the computer." This brings up a few questions. Is the parent using electronics as a more modern learning tool than a book? Is the parent directly engaged with the child during this attempt at learning? Are the electronic devices taking the place of direct interaction with a person, as a sort of electronic substitute teacher? Or is the television or computer just a plaything, or even a babysitter that allows the parent to engage in another activity?

Can electronics teach young children? Children under age 2 learn better from *live* presentations than from videos and are also more likely to remember information that is presented live. This suggests that interactions from people are better for young children, even when the information is well chosen. Watching cartoons or other programs that are geared for entertainment are not likely to be educational. Just as importantly, products such as *Baby Einstein*, which have been marketed as important for a child's learning, have no proven effectiveness.

I have started with the best-case scenario for electronics- the computer or television as teacher. What about the effect of screen time for play or entertainment? Watching television or a computer significantly reduces the time a child spends interacting with other children or adults. Heavy television viewing families read less, and children in these families are more likely to develop reading delays. In general, young children who watch more television are at risk for delays in development.

Background television is surprisingly harmful. Adults in these homes spend less time talking to their children. Being *spoken to* is strongly associated with learning language. Background television also shortens the time that a child will play, and lowers a child's focus while playing, due to repeated distractions from the screen. This is true even for programs that seemingly may not be of interest to a child.

While I am referring to young children in this discussion, there is a wealth of research about older children and television viewing. The negative effects range from shorter attention spans, to increased risk for obesity, to increased aggression when exposed to violence.

To put the latter bluntly, if your son is aggressive, watching *Power Rangers* and *Teenage Mutant Ninja Turtles* is not going to help him.

Finally, we should all remember one of the basic lessons of media education: "All media messages are constructed." Most of this construction is to build wealth, not a solid foundation for your child. As parents, we are the guardians of what will shape our child's worldview. It is essential that we supervise them, and limit their media exposure, so that children do not become the victims of mass marketing, and educational and social deprivation.

k.   Eliminate the word bored from your dictionary

Let's face it. We all have certain things that set us off. For me, the words, "That's boring" are right up there. In my usual smart-Alec manner, I usually reply, "I'm sorry. I didn't understand. I think you may have used a b-word that causes a force-field between us." It's better than getting upset.

We are blessed these days with a wealth of ways in which we can be entertained. Perhaps this is as much a curse as a blessing. Sometimes we have so many choices that we take them for granted and we expect this luxury to last. Many parents feel like they cater to their kids, only to hear complaints when there is a brief lull. As the saying goes, "No good deed goes unpunished", or perhaps in this case, "No gift goes unprotested."

Older generations bemoan children who are unable to self-entertain. I guess this is understandable in times when the radio or phonograph was considered exciting. Old-fashioned mind games such as *20 Questions*, *I Spy*, and *Hangman* helped to pass idle time. Board games like *checkers* and *Monopoly*, and card games were staples around any house. People wrote letters. And most importantly, they had *down time*.

Most people of my generation can remember picking dandelions or laying on their backs, looking at clouds for fun. These activities, if you can call them that, served a few purposes. First, there was a mental health benefit-they allowed us to slow down and unwind. Second, they allowed our brains to become uncluttered, and in a position to imagine and create. If you are skeptical of this, investigate how today's leading innovative technology companies give their employees scheduled down time. Finally, they passed time and kept us from becoming, yup... bored.

As a parent of young children, you can set the stage for staving off boredom. You can start early with games like peek-a-boo. Hide a common item for a toddler and then go on an *adventure* to find it. Teach them *X's and O's* while waiting for the doctor, or draw pictures on the table paper. And most of all, read to them. Not only will this educate them and expand their language skills, it will show them ways to easily occupy themselves. If you are up for it, make up your own stories and tell them to the kids. Many years later, they will have fond memories.

Because, as one of my favorite kindergarten teachers says, "If you're bored, you're not using your imagination."

1.   How to manipulate your mother

The second most underrated sign of an infant's intelligence is his ability to get himself in trouble. Example: crawling towards the stairs is fun. This is only surpassed by the ability to manipulate his mother. Example: If I make a move toward the stairs then look to see if Mommy notices, she will chase me there. In my opinion, simultaneously getting in trouble and having your mother chase you is the coup de grace of baby smarts.

How are they so darned good at pulling our strings? I think the first factor is that babies are always learning. They are little sponges, soaking up information at an amazing rate. Much of what they are absorbing goes unnoticed by us, because we are consumed by *more important* issues. Part of what babies learn by observation is the behavior that gets their parents' attention.

The second factor is that getting our attention matters to them. This surely has something to do with social development at a very basic level, although I have no idea how the brain teaches them this. Somewhere along the line, evolution taught us that getting attention leads to being nurtured, both physically and emotionally. I suppose that makes it easier to understand when older kids and adults go overboard in the attention seeking department- they are just filling a basic need for nurturing.

Putting together the need for attention with the powers of observation is how they demonstrate intelligence. In the end, it comes down to trial and error. Which behavior gets Mommy to chase me? The actor, Dustin Hoffman, has said that finding the right way to deliver a movie line is like playing the keys of a piano. You keep trying different ones – do, re, me- until you get to the one that just sounds right- fa, so, so, so, so, so! When you hit it, you know. The same goes for babies. I imagine their little minds churning: Crawl here, crawl there, crawl for the stairs. That's it- the stairs!

As he gets older, and his behaviors get more sophisticated, so does his ability to manipulate you. "Tugging on her leg seems to work best when while she is on the phone." "Throwing a fit for Mom in front of Grandma seems to get me what I want the best."

Although I imagine these little thoughts going through a kid's brain, the amazing thing is that in all likelihood it rarely reaches their consciousness. It just comes naturally.

Why do mothers receive the brunt of these behaviors? It is a sort of *left-handed* compliment. First of all, there is no one who seems to care so much when children misbehave. No one loves a baby more than his mother. Because you care, the reaction that a mother gives tends to be the most vigorous. It gets the most attention for him. When you add in that he *wants* his mother's attention more than anyone else's', the behavior begins to make sense.

Some children grow up into adults that bring manipulating their moms to an art form. Our cousin, Mark, has been doing this his entire adult life. He most recently asked his mother if she thought it would be okay to send a funeral flower arrangement to his aunt and uncle's fiftieth wedding anniversary celebration. Of course, she bit. "Jesus, Mary and Joseph, you can't do that, Mark!"
"But, Mom", he protested. "The flower shop is having a big sale."

In other words, if your child looks for you when crawling for the stairs, you may look forward to attention for many years to come.

Chapter 7: Skin and bones

a.   Moisturize, moisturize, moisturize

A baby's skin is a beautiful thing, but it is not always a pretty thing, much to a mother's chagrin. At birth and shortly after, the skin of some babies will develop impressive, pink bumps and blotches that last just two or three days, and are harmless. Early babies are often covered with a cheesy material called vernix. Many babies will develop a scale on their scalp known as cradle cap; this does not bother the baby, and responds well to baby oil before the tub, followed by a gentle flaking off of the crust with a toothbrush.

Children born past their due date will often have dried and cracked skin, which will be shed within a couple of weeks, like a snake sheds its skin. I tell parents that for the turkey to be properly cooked on the inside it has to be a little crispy on the outside. When this resolves, it is often replaced at about 1 month by a temporary outbreak of acne. All of these conditions are of little importance to the baby. But the most troublesome skin problem for many babies is persistent dryness.

Itchiness and irritation are what elevate dry skin from a nuisance to a significant medical problem that doctors call eczema, or atopic dermatitis. Eczema is an allergic inflammation of the skin. Dermatologists describe eczema as "the itch that rashes", meaning that the scratching is what leads to a lot of the redness. While young babies can't scratch themselves in a coordinated way, they can be seen to wriggle around uncomfortably, rubbing their bodies against their surroundings.

Older children and adults tend to get eczema in the creases of elbows and knees, but for infants, the face, scalp are more affected, as are the areas between the creases. If your baby has cradle cap that seems itchy, and instead of resolving within a couple of months, it worsens and spreads to other areas, it might actually be eczema instead. Again, regular cradle cap is not itchy.

Just like other allergic conditions, such as asthma or hay fever, it is difficult to cure eczema. As in these conditions, you will have more success and less frustration if you treat it like a chronic condition, and have a plan that you can use and adapt, depending on how your child is doing at a particular time.

The first step in treating irritation, in general, and eczema, in particular, is to avoid contact with irritating products. We generally suggest staying away from perfumes and dyes of all kinds, including soaps, laundry detergents and moisturizers. In severe cases, her clothes may need to be washed separately and double rinsed. Stick with non-irritating clothing and one brand of diapers that she seems to tolerate. A washcloth is better than disposable wipes for most changes, but if she is poopy, you can rinse the wipe under water before you use it.

Dove is a tried and true soap, where as *Ivory* has great advertising of a baby, but not as good performance in the minds of any dermatologist to whom I've ever spoken. More recently, there are many other more expensive products available. It is just as important is to limit the *amount* of soap. Aside from their diapers, young babies just do not get that dirty. Using soap once a week on the body is probably enough. You can still bathe every day, but in plain water. When you do use soap, most people like to wash first and then let the baby play in the bubbles. These kids should play first, then, if it is a soap day, do this, followed by a clean water rinse.

Trapping in moisture is the key to controlling eczema. This is where moisturizer comes in. Within reason, what you use is less important than how often you use it. Many good moisturizers are on the market. The cheapest is good old *Vaseline*, which is generically known as petroleum jelly. Some people shy away from this because it is greasy, but if a smaller amount is used, this becomes much less of a problem. *Aquaphor* is like *Vaseline*, but instead of a petroleum base, it is water-soluble, and accordingly more expensive. Again, *Cetaphil, Eucerin, Aveeno, Johnson & Johnson* and others all make good moisturizers. The key is that they be used

192

several times each day. If you keep one bottle of moisturizer at the change table, and another in your diaper bag, you can use it prior to every diaper change. For their day in and day out work, I refer to moisturizers as your work horse- they are not pretty or fancy, but they get the job done.

Think of avoidance of irritants, and moisturizer as the first two steps of your treatment ladder. The better you do with these, the less medication you will need. However, some babies will need medication some or all of the time. If moisturizer is the workhorse, hydrocortisone is the show horse- it comes out once and while a makes things look pretty. Over-the-counter strengths of hydrocortisone (0.5 or 1 %), are relatively mild, and can be used up to twice daily for problem patches. It is always best to use as little hydrocortisone as possible. Prescription strengths of cortisone can be prescribed by your provider, if the milder forms do not control his symptoms. If itching is a problem, *Benadryl* or other anti-histamines may be needed, but for young children, you should ask before starting these. Just like other conditions, there will be a large spectrum of eczema severity. A certain percentage of kids will need prescription strength medicine all the time; most will need it sometimes and others not at all.

You can climb up and down the ladder, from moisturizer, to steroid and back, as your child requires. I think of it in blocks of one week. For example, last week she was good so I only needed moisturizer. This week it flared up so I used 1% hydrocortisone twice per day. If next week is better, I can go down to once a day, and then back to just moisturizer.

And more moisturizer, and more moisturizer.

b. Leaves of three, leave them be… and a few others, too

It may seem like a discussion of outdoor health issues is premature in a book about young children. I might have thought so, too, had my Andrew, at age 18 months, not managed to find some poison ivy which was creeping under a fence, and proceeded to try to eat it. Suffice it to say that plants and bugs do not discriminate against age.

As a non-native New Englander, I developed a mild obsession with poison ivy after the Andrew episode with this plant (which ended uneventfully with the help of a few days of prednisone). Someone comes into my office on Cape Cod almost every day with poison ivy, unless the ground is covered by a foot of snow. Even then, kids still sometimes find a way to touch it. There is a patch in the woods about ten feet from my office's back door, which I pull back each year, wearing what resembles a space suit. Still, I keep enough for *field* trips, so that afflicted kids and parents can see it up close and personal, BUT NOT TOUCH IT!

Leaves of three on a vine with no prickers is a good way to start thinking about poison ivy, because this appearance is consistent throughout the warm weather season. Leaves sprout in the North in early May, and last until mid-October, and this will be earlier in warmer climates. A lot of people mistakenly look for *red and shiny*, but the leaves are only red when first sprouting, and in the fall, when yellows and oranges also occur prior to shedding. From November to April there are no leaves, but the vine and roots contain the same irritating oil as the leaves.

Not everyone is prone, but you really don't want to take a chance with your child. Avoidance is best. If he does touch it, throwing the clothes straight in the washing machine, and washing any exposed areas with soap and water as soon as is practical will reduce the exposure. Specialized soaps, such as *Tecnu*, are frequently used by landscapers, but there is no good research to suggest they work better than soap and water (1).

Once the rash starts, it is at least a two-week process, if left untreated. Home remedies include bathing in salt water and applying creams. I have never been impressed by *Calamine* lotion doing much other than causing a mess, but that is just one person's opinion. Any good cream kept in the fridge will soothe due to its temperature. Over-the-counter strength hydrocortisone can be applied, but is not strong enough to knock back this powerful dermatitis. When the face, genitals or extensive areas are affected, we usually resort to prednisone-type medication by mouth.

195

Prescription strength steroid creams can help less severe cases. However, by far the best treatment is to not get poison ivy in the first place, by careful scouting during outdoor adventures. This begins with you, as the parent, and can be passed on to your child as an important life lesson.

Now, maybe you live in a different climate, and poison ivy is irrelevant to you. I can guarantee, though, that another plant will be out there that causes contact dermatitis. What ever this may be- poison sumac, oak or even mangoes or lime- the same principles will apply. For young children, eating poisonous plants may be an even greater danger. These plants can be indoors or outdoors. Berries are attractive to young kids, but there are many other non-berry plants whose leaves can be poisonous. Mushrooms are also an issue: as my kids used to say, "Don't eat the mushrooms because you could get poison ivy." Full points for trying, at least.

It is impossible for a parent, or even for most doctors, to be experts in poisonous plants. There are a few simple things you can do to protect your child. First, watch your children closely. There is no substitute direct supervision. Second, avoid plants inside your house that are poisonous- your local garden store will know, and if not, the Internet has several good resources. Finally, if your child does manage to eat a plant, take a small cutting and put it in a zip-lock bag. Then, call poison control. If symptoms develop or if poison control is concerned, head to the local emergency room and bring the sample.

Do not give ipecac syrup. This old potion was used a lot in the past to induce vomiting after the ingestion of a poison, but it is now rarely used because it can get in the way of treatment that the emergency room might want to give.

Finally, a few quick words about kids with autism and developmental delays. In addition to the risks that all kids face, sometimes kids with these diagnoses will have a particular interest in eating non-food items; a condition known as PICA. These kids need extra close supervision.

Outdoor play with children is not as common as it used to be, and this is a shame. We want to encourage active lifestyles, as well as the enjoyment that can come from an appreciation of nature. This can lead to a lifetime of fun. Just pray that as your child grows up, and explores on his own, that he is not the one that wipes himself with poison ivy in the woods.

c. Sun safety is a life-long project

My father was always a beach-worshipper, if not exactly a sun worshipper. He has Mediterranean skin, and I don't recall ever seeing sunblock grace it. Then, at about the age seventy-five, he suddenly announced, "You know, I've heard the sun can be bad for your skin, so I think I'm going to stop tanning." I try hard not to laugh when he gets these sorts of revelations, but I probably didn't this time. In the end, I congratulated him, but needless to say, it was a little late to make this sort of a decision.

Sun protection should begin early, and continue often. For young infants, this essentially means complete avoidance of direct sun. New skin is completely vulnerable to burning, and has to be protected. Evidence now suggests that ultraviolet rays can cause skin damage as early as the first year of life (1). It can be a challenge to protect your baby's skin, while still getting outside for stroller rides, and the other activities that are good for your soul when you have a new baby. Sun-hoods on strollers and hats for babies are a good place to start, as are tents, but it is also important to be careful of reflected sun.

Sun block is misunderstood for several reasons. In general, it is a very good product, but there are significant limitations. First of all, almost none of the commercially sunscreens recommend their use under six months of age. This is not because they are unsafe. In other warm countries such as Australia, they are routinely used at an early age. Instead, it is probably because there is not enough money to be made in this age group to make testing financially worthwhile. Living in a beach community, I still advise people to stay out of the sun with their babies, but if there is an unavoidable situation, then sunblock is better than sunburn.

Sun Protection Factors, better known as SPF, are also subject to marketing. Dermatologists generally recommend SPF 30 or higher. SPF 30 generally blocks 97 percent of the sun's Ultraviolet B (UVB) rays. Increasing to SPF 50 only increases protection to 98 percent. These tiny increases in protection are accompanied by substantial cost increases. Remember, as well, that you can still burn with most high SPF sunscreens, especially in hot climates and where there is a lot of reflected light, like a beach or body of water. Finally, SPF only refers to the type of ultraviolet rays that the product protects against. In previous years, it was only UVB rays. Most sun blocks now protect against UVA as well.

The next misperception is that kid sunblock is a lot different than adult sunblock. Do not be surprised if your kid sunblock is just adult sunblock in a different bottle, which happens to cost more. Avoidance of irritants is a little more consistent in children's sunblock. Specialized products are now emerging, but are still in their infancy (yuk yuk). Just as when we discussed moisturizers, the general recommendation is to find a product that is perfume and dye free, that is well tolerated by your child, and that works well, and stick with it. Use more rather than pay more.

Finally, and most importantly, sunblock has now been shown to prevent skin cancer, at least in adults. It took a while for this evidence to develop, maybe because older sun blocks did not protect against UVA rays. Hats, sunglasses, and sun-protective clothing really are an essential and underused part of protecting your child highly. Sun-protective clothing is underrated and underused.

And do not forget how beautiful it can be at 8 am or 7 pm when the crowds are not at the beach or the park, and the temperature is pleasant.

d. Things that go bump when they bite

You don't like bugs. You don't like rashes on your child's skin. So, I suppose it comes as no surprise that you hate when bugs cause a rash on your child's skin. This is true whether it is a bite, or a sting, and even more so if the bug is burrowing. While most of these bug issues are just annoying, some are very uncomfortable. Occasionally, serious illnesses occur, and since the media love to publicize these cases, many people fear for their child's health. As usual, the best approach is to remain calm.

Mosquitoes are the most common insects to bite children. The distinctive small itchy welts in exposed areas are easy to recognize. Some people get really big welts; I refer to them as being *tasty*. A large local reaction is not more serious, just more itchy. Like any reaction, we only get concerned with lip swelling, tongue swelling and trouble breathing. Many mosquito bites can be prevented through long-sleeved clothing and by avoiding the outside at dawn and dusk. The best mosquito repellent is still DEET (diethyltolumide), which can be used safely as early as two months. Low concentrations of DEET (less than 10 per cent) are often recommended for children. We almost never recommend DEET strength greater than thirty percent (1). Studies of citronella and other insect repellents have shown disappointing results. Fortunately, most mosquito bites in the US and Canada are otherwise harmless. Occasionally, mosquitos can carry viruses such as *EEE* (Eastern Equine Encephalitis) and the West Nile Virus. These viruses are rare, and, provided that public health officials are doing their job with spraying programs and notification of the public, there should be no need for panic.

Flies and fleas cause similar problems to the mosquitoes. Bites from large flies often hurt, whereas small fly and fleabites tend to itch like mosquitoes. Fleas are most often thought of as coming from pets, but there are other common outdoor varieties, in places such as beaches. Bites on the ankles and lower legs of children old enough to walk are common, but crawling kids can get them more widespread. A good trick to see if you have fleas in your rug is to walk around in white socks. You should soon be able to see the small, black fleas on your socks. There are a number of ways to get rid of the fleas. If you need to flea *bomb* your house, it should be done when the children can be elsewhere for at least four hours. Do not apply more than is needed, rooms should be ventilated, and children prevented from crawling on *bombed* surfaces. More information is available at the National Pesticide Information Center (http://npic.orst.edu).

Bed bugs cause tremendous anxiety, and have recently become more common. Many people bring transport bed bugs to their homes after staying in hotels. Something about being bitten in your bed is disgusting, even though bed bugs do not carry diseases. They do itch, however, and tend to bite in a line of three, known as *breakfast, lunch, and dinner*. The itching and rash sometimes do not begin until a few days after the bites, which increases the chances of the bugs being brought to other locations in clothing, and suitcases. The best way to prevent bed bugs is a careful inspection of any bed outside of your own (2).

Bee and wasp stings hurt. There is usually no doubt about these ones, because there is instant crying, and you can usually see the bee as well. The discomfort can be treated with ice and with pain relievers. The main concern with bees and wasps is the possibility of allergies. Just like other potential causes of allergy, there are a few things that can happen. Most people will not be allergic at all. Some will have a local skin reaction with exaggerated swelling or hives. This kind is not serious and can be treated with antihistamines like *Benadryl*. If your child has a local reaction with a first bite, it is very likely that future bites would only cause a local reaction, and not a more serious reaction. The whole body reaction, with breathing difficulties, is the understandable fear of many people. It requires immediate attention. Once this occurs, a child should always have an epinephrine shot (*Epi-pen*) available. Allergy shots are very effective at desensitizing children to bees and

202

wasps. This can substantially reduce the severity of future reactions.

Spider bites depend very much on the spider. In general, spiders cause a reaction by the injection of a toxin into the skin. In northern climates, the spider species tend to cause minor reactions, mainly red welts one to two inches in diameter, which tend to hurt rather than itch. There is often a visible hole in the center, which can increase in size slightly, since that is the location of the toxin. Ice and ibuprofen are generally the only treatments needed. Most spider bites heal within a few days. In southern climates, spiders can be much more toxic. The brown recluse spider and the black widow spider are the most common poisonous spiders. These cause pain, fever and flu-like symptoms. There may be a blistered area in the center of the bite. Occasionally more serious symptoms develop, so if you suspect a black widow or brown recluse bite, seek medical attention, and if possible bring the spider in a clear plastic bag (As if, right?)

Tick bites are one of the least favorite topics for doctors in the Northeast, not so much because of how bad they are, as for how much hysteria they cause. Ticks that cause infections in people can either be from small ones, known as deer ticks, or from larger ones, known as dog or wood ticks. Different stages of the life cycle result in different sizes of tick, and a tick will also become bigger after a *blood meal*, so it is not a bad idea to bring a tick with you in a bag if you need to see the doctor. Deer ticks are best known for carrying the germ that causes Lyme disease. Lyme disease can show up with a number of different kinds of symptoms. Early Lyme disease usually appears as a flat pink ring-shaped rash known as a bull's eye, or as an illness with fever and flu symptoms. The ring rash can be hard to see, especially if is over an irregular surface like an ear. Other parts of the body can also be affected, leading to a droopy face, swollen joint, or irregular heartbeat. Part of the problem is that these small ticks often are missed when they bite.

Parents in areas where Lyme is common usually inspect their kids each night. Bath-time is a good chance to do this. It is important to look in the scalp and hairline, as this is a common location for bites. If a tick is found, it is best pulled out slowly with a pair of tweezers. It can be very hard to pull them out. A tiny piece of tick left behind does not increase the chance of Lyme disease and is no more dangerous than a small splinter. It is not worth digging up the skin to get out this last small bit. When a tick bite is known to have occurred, serious illness is rare because you can mark the calendar and then watch for either the ring rash or a fever with flu symptoms, but with no cough and cold. At this point, you can call the doctor. It is not worth treating with antibiotics just for a tick bite because the chance of side effects from the medicine is higher than the chance of Lyme disease. Those who are very concerned will sometimes have a Lyme test done about four weeks after the bite, but since Lyme tests are not a perfect science, this strategy commonly leads to borderline tests that are hard for the doctor to interpret.

Last, but certainly not least, are scabies and lice. These are similar bugs, with scabies affecting the skin and lice the hair. Scabies often will start on the hands, with a small bumpy rash that is extremely itchy, and which spreads throughout the body. The skin will look like it has been thoroughly scratched. Scabies can be difficult to tell from eczema at times. Doctors often try to locate the mite in a scraping which is examined in a microscope, but this is not easy. Scabies is relatively easy to treat with an over-the-counter product called permethrin, which can be used down to age 2 months. Clothing and linens need to be washed in hot water. Non-washable objects in close contact with someone who has scabies can be put into a green garbage bag for a week. These strategies make recurrences much less likely (3).

Lice, on the other hand, are usually easy to diagnose because bugs are seen in the hair. You can also see small white egg cases, known as nits, which adhere tightly to hair. However, they are notoriously hard to treat, in part because of the need to carefully remove the nits from the hair, and in part because resistance to lice remedies has developed, just like it has to antibiotics for bacterial infections. It is best for you to discuss with your provider or nurse, which lice treatment is recommended in your area. Sometimes a short haircut is still not a bad idea.

Finally, a story. Many years ago, I saw a child who looked like she had scabies. She had already been treated twice by other providers who also thought this was the problem. Since there had been no improvement, I thought it might be best to have the child see the dermatologist. When the dermatologist said that the rash was actually due to a form of eczema, I was very relieved not to also have treated for scabies. However, in the meantime, the father had gone temporarily insane. He was completely freaked out by the possibility of scabies, and not having any idea where it had come from, he threw out their entire furniture set. Needless to say, he was not happy to hear about the misdiagnosis. The moral of the story is two-fold. First, as a doctor, unless I see a mite with my own eyes, I tell people it looks like it is probably scabies. Second of all, I tell the parents, "I have been wrong before. Don't throw out the furniture!"

e. Is that bug bite infected?

It seems like a simple enough question, until you realize that two of the main signs of infection are redness and swelling, and that two of the main signs of an allergic response are also redness and swelling. So, how do you sort the out the difference?

The normal response to a bite is a good place to start. Mosquito bites are the most common source of confusion. Most people develop a small, pink, raised and itchy area at the bite mark. It will reach its maximum size about two days later and be virtually gone within four days. Bites that follow this pattern are generally nothing to worry about, even though some of us develop a much larger red area than others, due to a more intense allergic response.

On the other hand, an infection usually takes some time to develop. It tends to come on a few days later. In addition to being red and swollen, an infection is usually painful. Severe pain with a rash is always important to follow up immediately, on the rare chance that it is due to a severe infection. Some routine infections can spread on the surface of the skin, while others will become raised like a boil. In time, a boil will come to a head and usually have thick white drainage. It can also spread to local lymph glands, resulting in a red streak on the skin.

When I see a swollen bug bite, it has to meet these rules for me to feel comfortable that it is not infected:

1. Redness should peak at the right time; that is, about two days after the bite.
2. The bite should not be painful or tender.
3. There must be no white pus.
4. There must be no red streak.
5. There must be no fever.
6. Itchiness is reassuring but not essential.

If it does not meet these rules, I will treat it as infected. There will be times that I am extra cautious, such as a bite near the eye or elsewhere on the face.

Following these simple rules has been very useful over the years. I have been wrong at times when I do not stick to the rules. And remember, as doctors, we learn that no rule is perfect. If in doubt, get the bite checked out because some infections can be serious.

f. Flathead

If every cloud has a silver lining, then I suppose that it is only fair for the opposite to be true. Every great thing has to have a small downside. The "Back to Sleep" campaign has done a tremendous job at reducing Sudden Infant Death Syndrome (SIDS). In fact, SIDS continued to decline by 20 percent between 2005 and 2011 (1). This is due, in large part, to efforts at promoting safer sleep. There are two small negative aspects to infants sleeping on their backs. First, they roll over a little later. Second, some babies develop flattening of the back part of the skull.

Essentially, rolling over later is of interest mainly to pediatric specialists, be they doctors, psychologists or physical therapists. Think of a turtle on its shell. It requires a lot of torque through the hips for a baby to go from her back to her front. Compare this to rolling from belly to back, which requires a simple push (and avoidance of that pesky arm that gets caught under the body). Although babies traditionally were said to roll from belly to back at about four months, and back to belly at five, we now see both around five months. Less time spent on the belly tends to delay babies developing the shoulder strength they need for that push over. *Tummy time*, which I refer to as working out for babies, is important for babies to develop the shoulder and neck strength they need.

Good strength also helps to avoid a flat head. Think of the force of gravity coming down onto an infant's mobile skull. This force, over time, can remodel the bone. The remodeling can take on a number of forms depending on the head's position. We used to see this mainly in premature babies. Due to their weakness, premies are unable to move their heads like bigger, stronger babies. Their heads also tend to be disproportionately large for their bodies. Most often, they would turn their head to the side and develop long narrow heads. Neonatal nurseries now work to avoid this issue by taking care to turn a baby's head regularly.

Healthy babies who sleep on their backs can develop flat heads in a couple of ways. Babies with relatively *square* heads have a nice big flat spot at the back of the skull. They are prone to get flattening straight across the back of the skull. On the other hand, a lot of babies have a little more of a point at the back. These newborns will have two smaller flat areas, one on either side of the middle. One is usually flatter than the other, and this tends to be the position of comfort for the baby. Laying like this over months will push that side of the skull forward at the front, to make up for flatness at the back. The result is that the side that is the flat at the back will have a prominent forehead. The skull ends up taking on a parallelogram shape. The neck muscles can also become tight on the same side because the neck is always turned.

All this is possible because of the rapid growth of the brain in the early months after birth, and the fact that the eight main bones of the skull (four on each side), have not yet fused together. Most of this head shape change is in the first four months, but it does continue after this, albeit more slowly. The end result can be cosmetically undesirable, but it has absolutely no effect on the brain itself (unlike a few rare conditions where the skull bones fuse too early).

As with so much of pediatrics, prevention is the best way to avoid a problem. If your baby has a naturally square head with a flat area at the back, or if your baby has low muscle tone, the risk of a flat head is higher. You may want to talk to your doctor about raising the head of the crib higher than the feet (I'll spare you the physics, but this makes gravity less in play.) You can also begin tummy time early. New babies will not tolerate it for long, but you can do it briefly multiple times daily, stopping just before they begin to cry. Finally, you can use front packs and infant slings when the baby is awake, to avoid unnecessary time on the back.

For babies with one flat side at the back, regularly turn the head to the other side. At first, it may go right back to the flat side. That is fine. Before changing the baby, turn the chin towards each shoulder and hold it there for five to 10 seconds. This provides some quick physical therapy with minimal effort. When the baby reaches six to eight weeks, she will start being more interested in the environment. Position the baby so that she has to look towards the non-flat side to see the world, or to get a toy.

If an issue exists, the one or two month check-up is the best time to raise it. By four months, most of the flattening is done. It will slow down if you act then, but not as much as earlier. By four months, bouncy seats and saucers, as well as back packs can take the weight off of the back of head.

What about helmets to correct flat heads? These have become much more common in the past few years. Most doctors feel that they are a personal choice. Myself, I would not use a helmet for a mildly or even a moderately flat head, but you may feel differently. Remember that the decision you make is cosmetic, nothing else. And absolutely, still sleep the baby on her back, in a nice sparse crib.

g.   Walk this way

" Keisha trips a lot."
"Molly's feet turn in."
"Joey is bow-legged."

These are really common concerns, especially in the second year of life. Thankfully, almost all of these gaits reflect normal ways to walk. The key when it comes to a person's gait is being functional. In other words, does it work for them? Let's take a quick tour of the legs to help understand the issues.

In fact, let's start with the lower spine. The spine is important because the nerves which control the legs, originate from the lower spine. Babies who are born with lower spine problems can have issues with these nerves. We used to see a lot more spina bifida, where the lower spine did not form properly. This is rare now that women are supplemented with folic acid, preferably before conception. Once in a great while, a baby can be born with fibrous tissue tethered to this lower spine. These babies may develop exceptionally high muscle tone in the legs, and have trouble with walking. In it's mildest form, tippy-toe walking can develop. Most toe walking is not as serious as this, but it should be checked out.

Normal hips will be flexed up and turned out at birth, giving the standard frog-leg appearance. This makes sense when you are squished inside your mother. After birth, they gradually relax and straighten out. Your baby will be checked carefully at birth to make sure the hips feel normally in the joint. An occasional baby can be born with a hip out of socket; this occurs especially in breech (butt first) babies. Do not be surprised if an ultrasound is recommended to check the hips out. Early detection leads to great results. Late detection can cause a lot of problems. If one leg seems longer than the other, this should definitely be mentioned early.

The hips of toddlers have a tendency to turn out, although turning in can also happen. If you want to know how your toddler's hips are aligned, stand him up and look at the kneecaps as if they were eyes. When the hips are neutral or straight, the kneecaps will point straight ahead. When the kneecaps point away from each other, the hips turn out. When they point towards each other, the hips turn in (I call this lazy eye of the knee cap.)

Other than the above, the knee joint itself does not figure that much into alignment, because the knee is a simple hinge joint. However, the angle the tibia bone makes with the knee does matter. If the upper tibia bone is rotated as it meets the knee, the tibia bone will turn in along its length. This makes the feet point towards each other, and is called internal tibial torsion. Many lay people call this pigeon toed. Turning in of the feet is seldom a serious problem. We no longer recommend special shoes, bars or the like to fix this. First of all, the treatments were unnecessary. Second of all, they didn't really work. My teachers used to tell patients that the fastest sprinters were pigeon toed. I don't know if this is really true, but it sounded good at the time.

If the hips turn out and the tibia turn in, it gives the illusion of bowing. If you are shown where the turning takes place, it can be very reassuring. True bowing is a bend in the bone. It was common in the days of rickets due to severe vitamin D deficiency. Thankfully, it is very rare anymore. Occasionally, the doctor will take an X-ray to make sure that the bones themselves look fine.

The ankles and feet are the most ignored part of this equation. A lot of kids have relatively flat feet. Flat feet in themselves are harmless, but in severe cases they can interfere with a toddler's walking. The bumps on the inside part of the ankle will almost touch in this case. As they child gets older, a good arch in the shoe will help a lot. Once the foot has finished growing, a custom orthotic is often used.

With feet and ankles, flexibility is important. This means free movement of the various joints. You might see your provider wiggle the ankle and different parts of the foot from side to side looking at flexibility. Some babies have ankles which turn in severely and are stiff. These are true club feet, which need serial casting and surgery. Sometimes just the mid-part of the foot (the metatarsal bones) is stiff and turned in. This is treated with just casting.

Fortunately, the vast majority of turning in and out of legs is not serious and very functional. The only hard thing is convincing members of older generations that it is okay to walk this way.

Cue Aerosmith!

Chapter 8: A firm grasp on germs

a. Immunizations are so good that people forget the diseases

The words pediatrician and passion seldom occupy the same sentence. Except, that is, when it comes to child health, and especially when it comes to immunizations. Most pediatricians believe that immunizing children against infectious diseases is the single best thing that we do for children. If you had to choose between having a doctor visit with me and getting your immunizations, the immunizations should win hands-down.

Why do pediatricians love immunizations? There are two reasons. The first is that the diseases prevented by immunizations are serious, and sometimes fatal. Diphtheria, tetanus, and bacterial meningitis are universally fatal if not treated. Whooping cough has a 20 percent fatality rate in young children. Polio can cause paralysis, and rubella (German Measles) causes birth defects. Diseases such as measles, chicken pox and influenza were not usually serious in healthy children, but they were so common that some children would get it bad enough to die. Most parents have not seen life-threatening chicken pox, but most doctors older than 45 have, and this is why we recommend immunizations so strongly. Everyone hates seeing children die, but when a death occurs from a preventable illness, we take it personally.

The second reason for our passion is that immunizations work really well. Most immunizations are 90-100 percent effective in providing immunity to a particular infection (the whooping cough vaccine has one of the lowest response rates, about 80-85%.) (2) This effectiveness has led to the elimination of certain diseases in well-immunized populations. For instance, polio is now almost unheard of in North America. These achievements have been attained with an extremely low level of serious side effects.

If vaccines are so great, why has there been so much controversy about them? There are several explanations. First of all, we have done such a good job of reducing or eliminating vaccine-preventable diseases that the average person is not aware of the risks. You only have to pay attention to outbreaks that occur in populations that are not immunized to know that these risks still exist. Because people do not remember the diseases, many parents are not weighing risks against benefits. While doctors feel that the benefits far outweigh rare side effects, some parents only look at the risks. When a rare serious vaccine side effect occurs, people may not realize that 100,000 kids have been protected, and many lives saved due to the same vaccine.

The media plays a significant role in presenting unbalanced stories about vaccination. It is generally much more newsworthy to speak of a rare complication than it is to speak of many who were protected and therefore had *nothing happen*. The media's willingness to widely publicize celebrities who made false claims about perceived risks of autism from the measles-mumps-rubella (MMR) vaccine did a complete disservice to children. When these claims were unsupported by scientific evidence, that story did not get the attention it deserved. Even most good reporters are not scientists. They usually try to present both sides. But in science, evidence can prove that one side is right and the other is wrong.

Equally important is that most doctors do not understand the media. We are trained that we should be conservative in our promotion of a treatment. However, the Internet is far from conservative. Wild claims, based on a complete lack of science, can be made by anyone with a computer. The average person cannot be expected to know which claims are valid and which are invalid. The medical community has been unable to successfully reassure enough parents about vaccine safety, even though vaccines are extremely effective and safe.

The large number of vaccines that children are given at a young age also concerns parents unnecessarily. People worry that too many *substances* are being introduced into their child too soon. These concerns are understandable, but not founded in facts. Here is why: some old vaccines, such as the Diphtheria-Tetanus-Pertussis vaccine, were made from an entire cell's worth of proteins. Today's vaccines are much more pure. The entire immunization series of shots that a child receives, even though it protects against many more illnesses, contains fewer proteins than that one old DTP shot. So, a child is exposed to many less *substances*. As for the young age, it is really important to realize that babies are the most likely to get and by far the most likely to die from them most of these infections. It is essential to immunize babies at the earliest age possible. If I had my way, a baby would get one shot for everything before leaving the nursery. Unfortunately, that technology does not yet exist.

As for additives, such as mercury, aluminum or whatever else people are talking about on-line, just forget about them. Most vaccines have had mercury removed to appease the public, even though the amount was not considered harmful. The amounts of other additives are very small, and I would recommend focusing your energy elsewhere.

Bottom line: I vaccinated my children and you should, too.

b.   Your child's fever will not cause brain damage

"My child has a fever." This is the phone call which dominates a pediatrician's nights on call. Nothing inspires anxiety like a good old-fashioned fever- and yet, most of the time, the illness causing the fever is not serious. I like to use the term *fever outside the box* to help understand when to be more concerned.

For clarification, doctors consider fever to be a temperature greater than roughly 100.5 degrees F (or 38 C) rectally. This does not mean you have to take the temperature rectally, except in infants. The old teaching to add a degree to an underarm or other method of taking the temperature is not accurate- all we know for sure is that your internal (rectal) temperature is somewhat higher than the other routes. Doctors are not big on ear or forehead thermometers and we will not be concerned if you tell us that your child *runs low* and that 98 is really a fever for her (unless she has a severe neurologic disability). Feeling a forehead with the back of your hand is accurate if it feels fine, but not if the child feels warm- it just tells you to measure the temperature. Tenths of degrees matter in infants 3 months or less, because young babies are not always good at generating fever, and so these babies need a rectal temperature if there is any doubt. For older kids, tenths of degrees are not important, so the route of taking the temperature is also less important, as long as it is consistent. With the exception of young infants, if your child is not sick enough for you to allow a rectal temperature on yourself, then I would probably spare the child, too.

Most fevers are caused by routine viral illnesses. The fever generally starts near the beginning of the illness and lasts two to four days. Some fevers are higher than others. Some are persistent; others come and go, and are higher in the evening. Some fevers can easily be brought down with fever reducers, while others cannot. All of these patterns are okay, provided the child is otherwise behaving reasonably. Reasonable behavior means taking enough fluids to pee two to three times per day, breathing comfortably, and showing enough energy to be comfortable as a *couch potato* (or lap potato for infants and toddlers). Anything more than this is a bonus. Most kids with fevers are not very interested in eating.

With this in mind, it is easier to know what is not all right. For starters, if your child is 3 months old or less, and has a rectal temperature of 100.5 or higher, you need to call the doctor, even if it is the middle of the night. Do not give her acetaminophen (*Tylenol*) without a doctor's instruction. Babies at this age need to be assessed to see if they have a serious illness. Expect the doctor to want to do tests. In the first month or two, this will include blood tests, a urine test, and a spinal tap (removal of fluid from the lower part of the spine to test for meningitis). At this age, we take a *test first* approach to make sure that a young baby does not have a serious illness. Although it will seem scary, this is routine, and safe, and it is something that pediatricians do regularly.

Once a child is out of the early infant period, it will be much easier to tell when an illness is more or less serious. My three key questions over the phone are about general appearance, breathing, and hydration. Most parents consider their febrile child to be lethargic. For doctors, true lethargy is more than the couch potato I described earlier. It would be things like being unable to stand (provided she is old enough), not waking to feed, or not caring if I theoretically were to poke her for a shot. Obviously, we don't want you waiting to call until the child is almost comatose; the point is that I am not concerned by mild reductions in energy. Breathing is somewhat easier to judge. A lot of kids with fevers will breathe shallowly and a little quickly to *blow off* the fever. It is not normal to work hard when breathing, which means using your chest and neck muscles such as you would after sprinting around a track.

Dehydration comes on in stages. It happens much more quickly when there is vomiting with the illness than when there is just poor intake, or even diarrhea. If your child is not vomiting, dehydration seldom occurs in less than 24 hours unless extreme conditions such as a heat wave exist. The first thing you will see is a mild decrease in peeing; healthy kidneys recognize the need to hold on to the body's fluids. After this, the heart rate will increase and eyes and lips will become dry. Many people talk about a young baby's soft spot *sinking* when dehydration occurs. In almost 25 years of caring for children, I have not been able to become reliable at determining this, so I would not expect this of you.

Notice that I have barely mentioned the height of the fever. This is much less important than what we have already discussed. You can be very sick with a low fever and not that sick with a high fever. You do not have to panic if the fever is over 104. You do not have to rush to the Emergency Department either. Grandma was right almost everything, but not about high fever causing brain damage. This idea probably dates back to a time when we did not

221

understand the cause of many infections. We now know that how the child is acting is much more important than the number on the thermometer. Although every child will look better when the fever comes down than when febrile, there are definitely degrees (excuse the pun) of how sick a child will look with the fever. If he looks sicker than you think is okay or are not sure, then call.

The pattern of the fever over days is more important than the height of the temperature at any one moment. For example, if you are 101 one day, 103, the second day and 104 the next, you are still heading into the illness, whereas the opposite pattern usually means that you are starting to improve. This is the main use for taking the temperature, not the change in temperature from hour to hour. In other words, it is also okay if the fever does not come down right away. On the other hand, fevers that last longer than four days have a higher chance of needing medical treatment. If the fever has not broken by this point, it is time to see the doctor.

This brings us to treating the fever itself. If I have convinced you that the fever itself is not dangerous, you can start to understand that the main goal in treating fever itself is to improve comfort. Doctors still debate the purpose of fever and whether the fever serves a role in fighting infection. I have not met too many parents who care about this when they sense that their child is uncomfortable. Since treating fever usually makes a child feel more comfortable, most of us lean towards treating it.

The two medications we heavily rely upon are acetaminophen (*Tylenol*) and ibuprofen (*Advil, Motrin*). Aspirin should not be used anymore to treat a child's fever because it can lead to a rare, serious disease called Reye's Syndrome. If you ask 99 pediatricians whether to give acetaminophen, ibuprofen, or alternate the two, you will probably get 100 different answers. I will try to explain the different approaches. As I mentioned above, under 3 months of age we do not want you to use either without consulting your care provider. Between 3 and 6 months, use acetaminophen because ibuprofen is not approved for use in this age group. Over 6 months is where the differences in approach begin. Acetaminophen is a very well tolerated medication (in appropriate doses); however, it is not quite as effective a fever reducer as ibuprofen, and acetaminophen lasts only about four hours. Ibuprofen is a better fever reducer and generally works for six to eight hours; however, for some people it causes stomach upset and can occasionally cause stomach irritation.

Some providers like acetaminophen; others like ibuprofen. Some will say alternate the two, giving the acetaminophen no more than every four hours and the ibuprofen no more than every six hours. This latter approach is the most effective at keeping the fever down, but the trade-off is that it means giving more medication. A few providers will say don't use any medication at all because the fever itself is not harmful. Since comfort is my goal, I recommend the following. If the child is sleeping, he is probably comfortable, so leave him be. If he seems uncomfortable, I start with

223

acetaminophen, since it is the gentlest. If the acetaminophen is not effective, you can then try ibuprofen. I would hesitate to use ibuprofen if he is vomiting. If ibuprofen works but less than six to eight hours, and he is uncomfortable in between, this is the only time I recommend alternating the two. If neither is working, remain calm, since this is also not a good predictor of the severity of the illness. I seldom suggest baths for fever, whether *cool* or *tepid*, because most kids hate being bathed while febrile. They often scream, shiver, and turn colors that look really unpleasant.

What about seizures from fever? These can definitely occur in about 1 in 100 children between the ages of 6 months and 5 years of age. This tendency often runs in families. Fortunately, they are seldom serious, although as a parent you will probably feel like he is dying the first time you see one. I usually tell parents that he will never remember, but you will never forget. The problem with febrile seizures is they usually occur right at the beginning of an illness, often before you even knew he was sick. For this reason, fever reducers are not very effective at preventing recurrences. On the other hand, if you call and tell me that your child has had a 104 fever for 24 hours, I can almost always reassure you that he is in the 99 per cent that do not have febrile seizures, because it would have already occurred if he were prone.

If your child has a seizure, febrile or otherwise, turn him on his side. He will look like he is not breathing but that is okay. Do not stick anything in his mouth. If you are really composed, look at the time, so you can know how long it is lasting. Call 911 if it lasts more than five minutes; sooner if you live in a remote area where it will take longer to reach you. If this is the case, your provider will likely give you a medication you can administer for future events (which only happen in about 1/3 of children). If the seizure stops, and it has never happened before, bring your child to be seen. If it has happened before and is typical (brief, and involving the whole body), call your provider to make a plan.

As much as I try to reassure you on the subject of fever, you will still worry- we have all just been conditioned this way for too long. When my kids were little, despite Sandee's knowledge of the fever phone chat, she would still call to tell me that one of the kids was *burning up*. And as much as I would reassure her, when I arrived home, I would often get that same, worried feeling. Because what fatherhood taught me more than medicine, is that you are looking down at the most precious being in the world, and the thought that something terrible could happen is almost impossible to accept.

Fortunately, I have a good doctor to call when I am worried about my child's fever- my partner.

c.   How infections are spread

In about 1860, Louis Pasteur discovered that the growth of bacteria could contaminate milk. But it was several years earlier

225

that an Austrian doctor, named Ignaz Simmelweiss, figured out that it was unsanitary for doctors to go directly from the morgue to seeing patients without first washing their hands (1). Incredibly, his peers ridiculed him, but we now recognize that Simmelweiss was the first modern infection control specialist. One hundred and fifty years later, hand washing is still the key to reducing the spread of infections.

Infections generally go from one person to another in one of three ways. Most colds and flus are spread by *respiratory droplets*; these are tiny particles that contain a particular germ. We can cough these on each other, but more commonly they are present our runny noses and eyes. Stomach bugs are spread mainly by the lovely-sounding *fecal-oral* route. Just as it sounds, a microscopic particle of the feces of one person is touched by another, either directly or on food which is consumed. The third route is known as *direct contact*, which we see in skin and sexually transmitted infections.

The hands are to blame for spreading most infections. For colds, typically we touch our runny eyes or nose, and then touch something else. Another person then touches the object that we did and touches his or her eyes or nose. The virus is carried in this way from one person to the next. I read once that the worst thing you can do with a person who has a cold is play cards. The cards pick up the virus from one person and are transferred to the next one. Interestingly, you have a higher chance of getting a cold from shaking an infected person's hands than by kissing him.

226

The same is not necessarily true for stomach bugs. If you change the diaper or clean up the vomit or diarrhea of your infected child, and then miss a spot on your hands while washing, you now are in contact with the virus. You need only to touch your own mouth or a food item to complete the germ transfer.

Skin infections are a much bigger concern than was the case twenty years ago, due to the increase in bacteria that are resistant to common antibiotics. The best known of these is methicillin-resistant staphylococcus aureus, or MRSA, as it is usually called. These infections can be passed on by touching an open wound, or by touching a surface which an open wound has previously touched.

For all kinds of infections, the key to preventing spread is through good hand washing. As simple as it is, washing the germs of your hands keeps the germs away from your other parts. The more often and more thoroughly you wash, the less likely you will be to get sick. Studies have shown that hand washing effectively reduce the spread of infectious diseases and reduce school absences (2). The choice of hand cleanser is less important. Good old soap and water or alcohol based hand sanitizers are both very effective. Anti-bacterial soaps are generally not recommended because they do not evaporate from the skin and as a result, allow bacteria to develop resistance.

There is another part of infection prevention which is often overlooked. Since most infections occur through contact with the nose, eyes and mouth, we can prevent infections by learning to avoid touching those areas. This is harder than it sounds, because it involves everything from not rubbing our eyes when we first wake up, to not rubbing our nose when it is itchy. Still, if the germs do not make it to these entry portals to our bodies, they will not make us sick.

Needless to say, this is very difficult to teach young children. Infants and toddlers are forever putting things in their mouths. It takes a long time to teach a child to resist this urge. In the meantime, we can help by keeping their environments germ-free by cleaning toys at home and by avoiding public indoor play areas during flu season. Daycare is a whole other story, and I'll address this in a separate chapter.

A crack in the skin is also a crack in the door for germs. For children with skin conditions such as eczema, and for those of us who work in healthcare or childcare, good hand care is important to prevent infections. Repeated washing, and especially repeated use of alcohol-based products dry the hands, and make them prone to cracking. A good moisturizer can go a long way to keeping your hands healthy.

If you or a family member becomes sick, you can do damage control by trying to prevent the spread of infection to others. In the last few years, people have become much better about coughing into their elbows rather than their hands. Again, since hands touch other things, keeping the germs off our hands keeps the germs off of other objects. Kids as young as 2 can be taught to cover their coughs in this way.

Disposable tissues are better than old-fashioned handkerchiefs, which become a germ-infested mess. Tissues need to be put straight into the garbage and not left sitting around. An open skin infection should be covered so that sores do not touch surfaces and people. And with stomach bugs, repeated and thorough cleaning of toilets, bathrooms, clothes, diapers and hands is essential. If you have a second bathroom, quarantining the sick person in one room and having everyone else use the clean one can be very helpful, too.

This subject is not very exciting, but it is important. I have always wondered if Simmelweiss had obsessive-compulsive disorder. He certainly was not popular with his peers. But we have him to thank for keeping our children and ourselves from getting infections. And that is a big deal, because there is nothing worse than seeing our little ones feeling bad.

d. Daycare is germ heaven

If you were planning a place to optimize the spread of germs, it would be hard to do better than a daycare. It takes susceptible hosts who cannot control their own secretions, puts them in close contact with each other and lets them share many objects. Needless to say, many parents have felt the frustration of the recurrent illnesses which often go along with a first year in this environment.

I have dealt with many daycare owners over the years. Most are loving, nurturing, and obsessed with cleanliness. They want to keep the children healthy and they want to keep their facilities clean. Even with such good intentions, it is almost impossible to win the battle of infection prevention. If you think back to the previous chapter, and the factors that contribute to the spread of infection, almost all are present in a daycare. Young children do not just touch objects; they mouth them, drool on them and sometimes do worse things.

The numbers are against daycare providers- there are always more children than adults. These children are usually in a small space, especially in the winter. In a sense, this creates an over-crowded living arrangement. We know that close contact is a key factor for the spread of infections. In former days, over-crowding was a key reason for outbreaks of infection. In daycares, we have multiple children in one room, re-creating the kind of conditions in which infections can run rampant.

Most good daycares have strict policies about non-attendance while sick. Every time I see a child referred by a daycare with what appears to be minimal illness, I have to remind myself what they are up against. Even when children are excluded for illness, the best that can be done is damage control, because, as we all know, many illnesses can be spread before the child shows much in the way of symptoms. Excluding the child when illness becomes obvious is often too little too late.

Sometimes good intentions lead daycare directors to poor policies regarding antibiotics. Many lay people feel that it is better to see a child on antibiotics because this will make a child less contagious. Because of this, it is not uncommon to hear a parent say, "The daycare director says he can't return until he is on antibiotics." As we all know, antibiotics can be important for serious bacterial infections. However, too much antibiotic use can lead to the development of infections which are resistant to antibiotics, and as a result, more dangerous.

Here is how a daycare drug resistance problem occurs. When we ingest an antibiotic, it kills certain bacteria in our bodies. Ideally, this would just be the bacterium causing an infection. Unfortunately, this is not the case. Many bacteria that are living harmlessly, and sometimes cooperatively, within our bodies can also be killed. When harmless bacteria are killed, this leaves a void for other germs to take up residence in our bodies. These new germs are the ones which are resistant to the antibiotic that was used (otherwise they would not survive). This can be the basis for diarrheal infections such as C. diff, resistant skin infections such as MRSA, and other organisms which are resistant to common antibiotics. If only an occasional child needs an antibiotic, then there will not be a proliferation of these bacteria, but if kids have unnecessary antibiotics pushed upon them, the daycare becomes a haven for antibiotic resistance. The children then serve to spread around the germ, and the scenario can become potentially dangerous.

How can you, as a parent, hope to succeed in finding a healthy daycare environment in the face of all these germs? It is not easy, but a few tips can help. First of all, when looking into daycare, among your questions should be how many children are in the group together. More children means more germs. A good provider: child ratio is not only important for nurturing; it helps to supervise the children with respect to cleanliness, not to mention safety. Ask how often toys are cleaned. Ask what the policy is for exclusion of a child for illness, and if the daycare seems to promote the overuse of antibiotics, consider directing them towards the www.cdc.gov/getsmart website, which reviews this topic in detail.

e. Glands are the army barracks of the body

We usually like things to be smooth rather than lumpy or bumpy. A lumpy bed or lumpy gravy will not be very popular; nor will a bumpy ride. When it comes to our children, lumps and bumps take on a whole new meaning because, let's face it, most people are worried about cancer. Fortunately, bumps under the skin are not serious 99.99 percent of the time. The most common bumps are called lymph nodes, which are also referred to as lymph glands.

Think of the white blood cell as the basic soldier of the body. They protect us from infection and other kinds of inflammation. Although white blood cells are thought of as being in the blood itself, there is another body system which acts to collect fluid which has leaked out of blood, mix it with white blood cells and drain back into the blood stream. This second system is known as the lymph system.

If the white blood cell is the soldier, then the lymph node is the body's army barracks. Lymph nodes are generally small, pea or bean sized lumps that are positioned along the lymph vessels in various locations. Just as different parts of a country need different barracks to protect them, different parts of the body have their own lymph nodes- these include under the arms, in the groin, and in the neck. The tonsils are specialized lymph glands in the mouth, as is the spleen under the ribs on the left side.

It is normal to feel small lymph nodes in children, especially in the neck and groin. A normal node will be slightly soft and, like a mouse, it will *skit* away from your fingers when you try to grasp it The closer a node is to the skin, the more easily it is felt. One particular gland at the back of the neck, sits right on the base of the skull. Parents of infants will ask about this one at least twice a month. I tell them it could stay there like that until the baby turns my age, which is a long time.

In the past, many doctors have used the line, "I worry about the kids whose glands I can't feel, more the ones whose I can", the idea being that the glands form an essential part of the body's immune system. Personally, I don't like this explanation, because there are plenty of perfectly healthy kids whose glands I do not palpate. Having said that, there is definitely a range of normal gland sizes in different kids and locations. For example, the gland at the angle (or bend) of the jaw, is often significantly bigger than any other, and can normally be as big as a cherry tomato. Some kids have tiny tonsils, while in others, they can be quite large and still be fine. It seems like kids who are allergy prone also tend to have larger tonsils and glands in their neck, perhaps because they are fighting the chronic congestion.

Just as the army needs more troops when there is a disturbance, so the body needs more white blood cells, and an enlarged gland provides a larger barracks. Typically, a local disturbance, such as a bug bite or rash in one part of the skin, will cause the nearby glands to enlarge. A generalized problem, like infectious mono, will lead to enlarged glands throughout the body. These glands are called *reactive* lymph nodes, because there is nothing wrong with the gland itself; it is just reacting to a problem in the body in an appropriate way. When the infection or other problem resolves, so, too, will the enlargement.

Lymph nodes themselves can occasionally become infected. When this happens, the gland will enlarge, but instead of only mild discomfort as is seen in reactive nodes, this node will be red and very tender. This often requires antibiotic treatment, and so the doctor should be called. Infected lymph nodes can sometimes form a boil (also called an abscess) within the gland, which requires drainage. Fortunately, this is uncommon.

Because lymph nodes become enlarged in cancer, it is, at times, very difficult to be reassured. Luckily, pediatricians feel normal and reactive glands every day. It is usually very obvious that rare time when there is cause for concern. For example, cancerous lymph nodes can become hard, *fixed* or attached to the skin, and uncommonly large. There may be other more serious symptoms such as fever, night sweats, weight loss, bruising or pain. All of these will prompt us to do tests, and in cancer, these tests are usually clearly abnormal.

It is pretty easy for an experienced provider to tell which glands are normal, and which require investigation. If you have been reassured, this is a very good sign. Often times, providers will tell parents to *keep an eye on it*, and let us know if it changes. Since the nature of glands is to change, I feel like this can drive parents a little crazy. I tell them to ignore a normal gland, unless it jumps out as them as larger, in which case they should call. This way you don't spend every day staring at it looking for minor differences.

And if you need to have it rechecked each time you come in to the office, that's OK, too.

f.   Microbophobia

Just when you think you have invented a new word, a *Google* search explains that a guy named Grant Showerman used it a hundred years ago. OK, so let's call microbophobia a good, underused word. An irrational fear of germs, too small to see, has the same effect as any other irrational fear. It keeps us from calmly preparing, in an appropriate fashion, for any risks we may face.

At the time of this writing, the microbe du jour is Enterovirus D68. It is just the latest bug in a long line of critters which has had the nation in a state of pre-panic. Before that there was Swine flu, Bird flu, Eastern Equine Encephalitis, West Nile virus and SARS (Severe Acute Respiratory Syndrome). Thanks to the wonders of twenty-four-hour news, all of these viruses have at one point been catapulted from obscurity to public enemy number one. The notion that they are too small to see, lends them a sort of stealth threat, which is amplified by the serious nature that the infections can sometimes pose. The Swine flu was particularly memorable to pediatricians, mainly due to the absolute chaos that it caused to our offices. At times, the hysteria led to over one hundred calls per day to our three-doctor office. One parent even exclaimed, "President Obama said that I need to call you to get my child a Swine flu shot." My witty receptionist replied, "Well, you'd better tell President Obama to get us some vaccine because he hasn't sent us any yet!"

I encourage people to think of these viruses like they might think of the ocean. After all, here on Cape Cod, we all think about the ocean. We know that it has the potential to be dangerous. We know that it must be respected, and proper steps must be taken to remain safe. And yet, we do not all run around screaming, "Oh my gosh. It's the ocean!" This is because we can see what we are up against, and we have a basic understanding of how it behaves. We also have enough familiarity to reduce our anxiety.

There are some situations in life when we could do with a little more fear and respect. Car travel might be a good example of this. About 30,000 people die every year in this country in motor vehicle crashes. Even so, some states still have difficulties passing good seat belt laws. The general public 's lack of concern and awareness is probably because due to our over-familiarity with car travel. We have completed car trips safely so many time that we begin to believe this is a guarantee.

Going back to the ocean analogy, we all know that there are certain times when extreme caution and strong preparation is absolutely appropriate. When a hurricane is coming, there must be multiple measures taken to protect us. There are true hurricanes in the virus world, too. HIV has been one of those viruses. It appears that Ebola will be another. As of October 2014, there have been thousands of deaths in West Africa, and one death in the United States. I truly do fear where those statistics will be a year from now. And yet, from having faced many emergencies in a career as a physician, I know that fear is not the answer to the crisis. Irrational fear, and actions that result from it, will certainly take away from our response. Knowledge, preparation and maintenance of calm in the storm are the way we will keep the ship righted.

I also mean no disrespect to anyone whose life has been impacted by any of the conditions which are described above. Any serious consequence or even death from a viral infection can be a tragedy. This is especially true when it happens suddenly to a previously healthy person. To minimize the risk of these severe complications, we need increased awareness and education, rather than over-dramatization for the sake of television ratings.

There is no question that the media plays a large role in setting the tone for the public's response to public health emergencies. The government has to take these matters seriously, as well; all the time, rather than in a knee-jerk response to a crisis. Bureaucracy can be just as detrimental to the response to an infectious threat as it can be to a hurricane response. Emergency response is no easy task, as we have seen repeatedly. Proper training and readiness will make us all safer, as will sufficient budgets to research ways to prevent and treat these threats.

If a calm approach is taken, we can relegate microbophobia to the movie theaters, where it belongs.

Chapter 9: Breathe deep and heart beeps

a. Is it asthma?

This should be an easy question, but in reality, it can be difficult. Even the explanation that follows is not an easy one, but here is my best attempt.

As you know, asthma is essentially allergies of the lungs. If you could look down into the lungs of a child during an asthma attack, you would see a combination of narrowing of the breathing passages (known as airways), and inflammation (redness, swelling mucus etc.). In adults and older children, specialists can used breathing tests known as PFTs – pulmonary function tests- to measure the flow of air, and to see if it matches the pattern of an asthmatic. In young kids, these methods are not practical. We end up having to make a judgment based on the history of the coughing, and on what we see from examining the child.

For young children, diagnosing asthma is not an exact science. This can be difficult for a parent to understand. There is no quick and easy test for younger children which will allow you to say, yes, your child has it, or no, she doesn't. There is no number like there is for diabetes. In fact, there is a point at which everyone could cough or wheeze; some of us might only do it in a smoke-filled room, while others do it all the time. The same person might do it at different times depending on the environment. There has to be a line drawn somewhere, to say it qualifies as asthma. As providers, we define asthma as *three separate illnesses that involve coughing and wheezing*. To add to the confusion, some asthmatic children do not wheeze, but have a history of repeatedly prolonged coughs. Sometimes we even give asthma medication, even though we are not yet calling it asthma; this can happen, for example, if it is a first or second episode of wheezing, and there is a family history of asthma or allergies.

There are other problems with the diagnosis. As doctors, we sometimes hedge on using the term asthma. You will hear things like *allergic bronchitis, reactive airways disease* and others, which all really mean the same thing. There are good reasons for hedging. First, the range of symptoms in asthma is so big that we fear you will think that your child has severe respiratory problems when it might be a very mild condition. In addition, using the word asthma can have serious implications outside the medical world: with life insurance and ability to pursue certain careers, such as the military or aviation.

Another problem occurs because the symptoms often improve as a child reaches the school age. Many times, parents will say that their child has *outgrown* the asthma. All of these issues may be going through your provider's head at the potential time of diagnosis (without you being aware). As providers, we need to be clear with you about where your child stands, but it can be complicated.

If the word asthma is used for your child's breathing, it can be helpful to ask whether the provider feels it is mild, moderate or severe. Remember, that asthma treatment has improved a lot in the last 25 years. And remember that the *a-word* is just a word. If your child walked into the office with a nuisance cough, that is also how she is walking out.

b. We should treat asthma more like we treat diabetes.

You probably know someone who has diabetes. If you do, you have seen that good diabetic control is all about trying to keep the blood sugar level as close to normal as possible. Diabetic educators show adult-onset patients how to reduce the amount of medication they might need- things like healthy eating choices, weight loss and exercise. They find the right amount of medicine (such as insulin) to take for everyday life, and then spend a lot of time teaching how to handle various situations that arise. They then teach how to adjust medication doses to *anticipate* what to do in the event of illness, vigorous exercise, or eating out at the buffet. This is a great model for how to manage a chronic (long-term) disease.

Asthma is one of the most common pediatric chronic diseases, and yet, many times we do not do it justice in terms of applying the *chronic disease model* in its management. We have already talked about the difficulties in establishing the diagnosis. It is worth talking about different aspects of asthma care to see how we can do better.

We are pretty good at preventing symptoms. A good asthma history involves learning *triggers*, or things that bring on symptoms. The two universal triggers for asthma symptoms are exposure to cigarette smoke and common colds. Others include pollen, dust, mold, pets, foods, exercise and temperature changes. These can usually be sorted out by just talking to a parent; not all kids need to be allergy tested. I usually save allergy testing for times when there is a serious issue, or when common-sense prevention and treatment have not been successful. Once you know your child's triggers, you can work on avoiding them. This is easy to say, but can be difficult to do: pollen can be everywhere, pets can be beloved, and no one ever said it was easy to quit smoking. In this sense, an asthmatic has the same struggles as a diabetic who is trying to avoid certain foods.

Asthma sick visits or *attacks* are also handled well by most providers. Parents do not need convincing to seek care when a child is short of breath. Providers are very good at settling down symptoms in the short term with medications, whether at the office, or the hospital, depending on the severity. The vast majority of symptoms can be improved with two medications groups. The first group is for temporary relief. This group as known as the *bronchodilators* because the medicine temporarily opens up the airways. Albuterol is by far the most common bronchodilator. The second group is the medicine known as *anti-inflammatories,* which as the name suggests, gradually reduces inflammation over time. These are usually some form of steroid (the anti-inflammatory kind, not the weight lifter kind).

Anticipating or predicting asthma attacks is generally not done very well. So often, a child will present to the doctor at the end of a cold, after a visit to Grandma's cat, or shortly into pollen season. Most of these asthma attacks are preventable. Providers need to take a more active role in this process. When the diagnosis of asthma is made, it is worth taking the time to figure out which triggers affect your child. As a parent, you should ask your provider for help with this. Understanding and acting on the triggers allows for much better control of the asthma.

Here is where the diabetes model can be helpful. If a diabetic is sick, is exercising or going out to eat, she is taught to adjust the medication *before* a problem occurs. Providers would scold a diabetic who repeatedly said, "Oh, guess what? My blood sugar was high after that ice cream." And yet, it is common for asthmatics to flare up repeatedly after a cold, when the flare is just as predictable. Every parent of an asthmatic should know when to adjust his child's medication in anticipation of an asthma attack.

The strategy will vary depending on the child. The mildest of asthmatics may only need to use albuterol for symptom relief. Albuterol treats symptoms temporarily; it does not prevent an attack from progressing. If albuterol is needed more than twice per week, other treatments are needed. These can be easily spelled out with the use of a written *asthma* plan. Simple asthma plan templates are available to document exactly how your provider suggests you act when asthma flares, and also at times when you learned to anticipate that it would flare. Smart parent/provider teams will act before the stressor occurs-for example, a week or so before pollen season begins, or prior to a visit to Grandma's (if she insists on keeping the cat). With colds, we suggest starting at the first sign of symptoms.

No one pays attention to the things that do not happen because of a well-designed prevention plan. Prevention is usually boring, but you really do not want your child's asthma to be interesting.

c.   The term *innocent heart murmur* should be replaced.

An oxymoron is defined as two adjacent words or phrases that seem to be a contradiction, such as efficient government, or favorite taxes. Innocent heart murmur falls in that same category. Let's talk about the heart so that we can better-understand murmurs and then discuss another term which might be more appealing.

Blood circulates to carry oxygen to the body's tissues and then return to the lungs for more oxygen. The heart is the pump. When blood flows smoothly, it is quiet; when there is turbulence in the flow, noises are made. Turbulence is usually present when blood is flowing from an area of higher pressure to lower pressure, often through a narrow opening. These noises are the basis of murmurs. The average person thinks of a murmur as being abnormal. In fact, this is only the case about 10 percent of the time in children. Abnormal murmurs tend to make a *whishing* sound, something like a washing machine, or a kink in a hose. These murmurs in children generally result from one of three situations. The most common abnormal murmurs are from small holes in the wall between the right and left sides of the heart. Narrowed heart valves will also cause an abnormal murmur, as will narrowing of a blood vessel. All of these situations share turbulent flow from high to low pressure through small openings.

On the other hand, 90 percent of murmurs occur in perfectly healthy hearts. These are generally due to high flow in normal blood vessels that occurs because a child's heat beats faster than an adult's heart. For this reason, the term innocent or flow murmur is used. Innocent murmurs sound like a cooing dove or a hooting owl.

Although I just said it, did you realize that innocent murmurs are normal? If not, it may be because the word murmur has been associated with disease, no matter what adjective we use to modify it. This is not just a pet peeve; literally millions of people believe their children have heart disease because of the perception of the word murmur. Studies have shown that even the mention of this word can have a permanent negative effect on how a parent perceives his child's health (1).

Cardiologists should have a better word than murmur for a normal sound. Since they do not, I have been brainstorming to come up with a suggestion. I thought about the dove and the owl, but a coo coo or a hoo hoo really didn't come out right! After many other inappropriate candidates, and some help from my co-workers, I would like to suggest that the term *innocent murmur* be replaced with the term *heart music*.

Music is not only normal, it is pleasant. It is full of life, just like the beating heart of a normal child. It does not sound serious; it sounds joyful. And as parents, we won't still be worrying about it 50 years later. It is possible that others have used this term before- it seems intuitive. Some cardiologists have definitely referred to the heart making musical sounds, but to my knowledge (and an Internet search), no one has adopted heart music as a formal term. I think they should.

In the meantime, if your doctor says your child has a murmur, ask if the heart is normal. She may say yes right away, or say that tests are needed to clarify the sound. If she says yes (right away or eventually), do not think disease. Think music. And do not worry at all if he wants to run around and make more.

Chapter 10: Eyes, ears, mouth and …

a. Is it a cold? Or her ears? Or teething?

Which parent has not asked this question in the middle of the night, when the baby will not sleep? In fact, it can usually be figured out with a simple method. I hesitate a little to give this explanation because, honestly, I have never seen it tested in a study- it would be nice if someone would. So, you are relying on practical experience. My other hesitation is that it may put me out of business by reducing the number of false alarm visits parents make.

The main problem is that the symptoms of teething, upper respiratory infections (which I prefer to call *common colds*) and ear infections overlap considerably. Each one can cause fussiness, poor sleep, reduced feeding and a congested or runny nose. All can also cause tugging at the ears- this happens because the ears, teeth, and throat are all served by branches of the same nerve. This is why our ears can feel pain when we have a sore throat. In a child too young to express himself, it can be difficult to figure out the problem.

I am more concerned about helping you distinguish ear infections from the other two problems, because we usually treat ear infections with antibiotics in young children. In other words, an ear infection is worth a visit to the office, while a cold or teething is only going to get you supportive care, such as pain relief, and reassurance. The only circumstance I can think of, where distinguishing a cold from teething is important, might be to know whether the child is contagious.

Teething usually starts between 4 and 12 months, although some babies bend these rules. The early teeth finish with the second molars, which usually break through after the second birthday-hence, the term two-year molars. Some kids get them one or two at a time; others in bunches. Some kids seem to suffer through every new tooth, while for others, the tooth is only discovered by looking. Some degree of nasal congestion can go along with teething, but teeth alone generally do not cause significant fever. Teething pain can be treated with cooled teething rings, pain relievers, (remember no ibuprofen under the age of six months), and occasional teething gel. Frequent use of teething gel can cause the baby to absorb too much of the numbing agent, and so this is discouraged.

We are all familiar with the common cold. Young children get the same symptoms as adults, namely sore throat, nasal congestion, cough, loss of appetite and sometimes fever, depending on the virus. Since these illnesses are caused by a variety of viruses, no specific treatment is available. The main goal is to provide fluids and comfort until she is feeling better. In addition to pain relievers, nasal saline (saltwater) drops can temporarily loosen up a stuffy nose. Sleeping with an elevated head can help post-nasal drip- this can be a challenge between the ages of six months and two, because the child is too old to stay still in a raised crib, but too young for a pillow. In older children, lemon and honey can relieve a sore throat. It is probably more important to remember *what does not work* for common colds- this long list includes Vitamin C, Echinacea, cough syrups and multiple other products. Vaporizers can loosen a congested nose- I prefer cool mist due to a lower risk of the machine becoming contaminated, and to avoid burns. Camphor rubs (such as *Vicks*), can be poisonous if ingested by a child and should not be used if this is a risk.

Ear infections usually follow a cold, teething, or allergic congestion. Think of it like this- becoming congested is like when a pond or pool stops flowing. If this water sits there long enough, it can become murky. Ear and sinus infections are similar to when the murkiness develops. This is the idea behind an ear or sinus infection leading to cloudy or green nasal discharge. However, green discharge does *not* always mean a bacterial infection, and does not always suggest the need for antibiotics, especially if the amount of discharge is going down. Green and getting better is getting better, while green and getting worse is getting worse. In other words, generally forget the green and just look to see if he is getting better or worse.

Some, but not all, ear infections will cause a fever. Fever at the start of a virus is common, but not a week later. Fever late in a cold always makes we wonder about the ears, although getting one virus after another can fool you. If a fever is the result of an ear infection, it is usually 102 or less. High fever is generally from another cause. And to add confusion, even young kids that get fever with their ear infections at an early age, usually stop doing so by the age of 2 or 3 years.

So, how do I make sense of this, and help you to make an easy decision. Here are a few rules that are not perfect, but usually reliable:

1. No cough equals no ear infection. In other words, if the child is fussy and tugging but is not coughing, it is probably the teeth. Exception: if there has been a previous ear infection within the prior month or two, the reliability of this goes down.

2. Fever of 101 or higher *at the end* of a cough and cold in a young child is an ear infection until your provider says it is not.

3. In between is in between. Cough but no fever could be any of the above and the only way to know is to look at the eardrum and the throat. This will keep your provider in business.

We have not talked at all about the treatment of ear infections, which is evolving over the last several years. For older children, most simple ear infections will resolve without antibiotics. For children under 3 years of age, this is not as effective, so an early visit makes sense.

And one last thing- even antibiotics will take from several hour to a couple of days to help. In the middle of the night, pain relievers are the way to go. This will keep you out of the Emergency Department at 3 am.

b.   Booger Nights

Cough, cough. Sneeze. Snort. Repeat.

We have all been through long nights with a cough. Watching your baby go through it is worse. Never before have you fully appreciated the value of being able to blow your nose. Young kids are too young to be propped up on pillows, and after about 6 months, too old to raise the head of the crib. You will end up spending a lot of time with them sleeping on your shoulder, and then struggling to make sure you do not doze off while holding the baby. Each time you try to lay her down, it will probably start again.

What can you do about this frustrating problem? Unfortunately, there are a limited number of options.

First of all, distinguish between a *sleeping* noisy, congested baby and an *awake, miserable*, noisy congested baby. The first group should be left alone, because the symptoms are bothering you more than him. Remember that what you see is more important than what you hear. In other words, when the chest is heaving up and down like a runner going around the track, this is the emergency. When the little guy snores like his grandfather, this is not an emergency. Remember that a baby's nasal passage is only about the size of the hole in a piece of macaroni, and it does not take much cheese to clog it!

If the baby is snoring but not coughing, the issue is almost certainly benign nasal congestion. Nasal congestion can interfere with feeding and sleeping. If the mouth is full or closed, it becomes hard to breathe out of the nose. Nasal saline drops can be used to relieve the congestion; these are available over the counter. A small *squirt* up each side will usually do the trick. When giving this, hold the saline bottle with your dominant hand. Cradle the back of the baby's head in your non-dominant hand, so that you can hold the baby's head a little higher than the body. This will keep him from gagging due to post-nasal drip. Hopefully, the baby will sneeze within a couple of minutes giving the saline (personally, I think this is why Mother Nature makes newborns sneeze.) If not, you can use a bulb syringe- this is a little, baby blue, rubber syringe that is a sphere on one end and comes to a point on the other. The pointy end has a hole. To use it, you squeeze the sphere closed, then insert the point in the nose and let the sphere re-inflate. This creates a suction, which helps to pull out boogers. Usually the ones you get at the hospital maternity ward are more effective than what you can buy in the pharmacy, because the pharmacy ones are so rounded at the sucking end that they don't go in the nose at all. Many parents worry that they will put the tip of the bulb too far. Common sense suggests that there is no need to go in more than ½ an inch. If you get brain tissue in the syringe, you went too far. Kidding. This will not happen.

Any of the illnesses associated with nasal congestion will have other associated symptoms, such as coughing, sneezing or fever. Cough causes the most grief. The cough from head congestion tends to be loose, which means that it sounds like there is phlegm being coughed up. A chest cough can be loose or hacking, like you might hear from a smoker. The cough that results from head congestion is usually from post-nasal drip, which means that phlegm is dripping out the back of the nose and down into the throat. The chest cough is either from phlegm coming up or from tickling the cough center without phlegm. Both of these coughs tend to be worse lying down, which is why nights can be so difficult.

In babies less than 4 to 5 months old, raising the head of the crib can help to lessen a cough. You are trying to get the head elevated up to 30 degrees, which is a lot. The old fashioned way is with books under the mattress. You can also buy wedges but these do not tend to create as big an angle. Ideally, you want the baby's head high enough that there should be a tendency for the baby to slide down into the bottom of the crib. This can be prevented by using a harness, which goes over the baby's sleeper like a diaper, and then is attached to the crib. Years ago, we used to use a small, thin blanket and the old-fashioned safety pins with the rubber protectors on the end to attach it to the crib. These days, ones with snaps or Velcro can be purchased on-line. It is important that the baby cannot slide off the wedge and become stuck. Once a baby is old enough to roll over, wedges become impractical. Unfortunately, between 6 months and 4 or 5 years of age, there is no good method to raise the head. Even 3 and 4 year olds will usually just roll off them once they are asleep.

Nothing makes me feel more routinely inadequate as a pediatrician than my inability to help kids cough less. When parents ask which medicine they should give their child, my answer is that if I had a good one, I would be sitting full-time on a warm island, drinking tropical fruit smoothies. Cold medication is an excellent example of how great marketing can be, while the actual products are dismally ineffective. There simply is no one great cough suppressant available. In fact, there isn't really even a good one.

For infants, we do not routinely give anything. Decongestants (the D in many products) can cause side effects in young children and should not be given at all. For children over two, honey can coat the throat and reduces cough at least as well as dextromethorphan (DM). There is almost no role for codeine-containing cough syrups. Expectorants, mucus thinners and other agents are essentially a waste of money.

Antihistamines such as diphenhydramine (*Benadryl*) can be helpful for coughs due to allergic symptoms. Sometimes the child seems to sleep better because of the sedative effect of the medicine rather than the reduction in congestion. As a general rule, you do not want to suppress a cough where the child is producing a large amount of phlegm from the chest. It is better for this to come up from the lungs. even if it is swallowed into the stomach.

Finally, a few specific coughs deserve special mention. Asthma is discussed in a separate chapter, but briefly the asthma cough tends to be deep. Most of the time there will be wheezing as well. Coughs that lead to vomiting can be from several causes. One of them is asthma; in the days before inhalers, doctors used to induce vomiting as a way to get the phlegm out. In fact, Teddy Roosevelt was given cigars to smoke for this reason! A very phlegmy cough can trigger gagging and can make a child throw up. The whooping cough (pertussis) occurs in prolonged bouts: cough, cough, cough, cough, cough, cough, cough, cough, cough… wretch and possibly then *whoop*. Croup is a narrowing of the windpipe, usually due to a viral infection, that leads to a barking cough. Once you recognize it, you can diagnose croup down the hall. Croup almost always comes on at night. It usually responds to keeping the child calm, giving humidity in the form of a vaporizer or steamed up bathroom, and bringing him outside. These days, we will often give a dose of anti-inflammatory steroid to reduce the windpipe swelling, and gasping sensation of a child with croup. Occasionally, if the gasping is persistent, it is necessary to go to the Emergency Department for treatment. You would be amazed how many kids arrive at the ED, looking so much better, because the cold night air has had more of a chance to work.

Last but not least, always remember to tell the doctor if your child choked on something. This is rare but when it happens, we need to know.

c. If you think your child does not hear normally, you might be right.

Ideally, every baby has a hearing test at birth. This means that babies who are deaf or hearing impaired can be diagnosed very early. This was not always the case. In the past, we waited until there were signs of delayed language skills or some other problem. It is not easy to pick out a deaf baby in the first six months of life. I even know pediatricians who were fooled for a while by their own child. Universal screening solves this problem, and early diagnosis allows for early treatment. Surgical implants in the cochlea of the inner ear provide these children an amazing opportunity to hear normally. It is remarkable to see what happens to a deaf baby after implant surgery. Their language literally explodes as the door of sound is opened.

After the newborn period, the most common reason for concern about hearing comes in children with frequent ear infections. You may be familiar with the feeling of *water* inside the ear. This sensation is due to congestion behind the eardrum, which doctors will refer to as fluid. At the onset of an ear infection, this fluid will be cloudy pus. After time, the fluid usually becomes clear, and then goes away. As an aside, water from the tub is not a problem. One of the jobs of the ear drum is to separate the inside world from the outside, and so bath water will not lead to middle ear fluid.

While the pus of an ear infection will usually clear up within the first week, the clear fluid can often take three to eight weeks to resolve. During this time period, a child will be prone to recurrences of infection. It is not unusual, for a child who gets sick early in the winter, to fight ear infections for several months. What does this hearing issue do to her language and development?

Surprisingly, the answer seems to be not that much. Studies suggest that children who undergo tubes sooner rather than later, do not seem to outperform the others on tests of language development. For this reason, we usually take a wait and see approach. Ear, Nose and Throat doctors usually suggest that infections which persist three months may warrant the placement of *tubes* in the middle ear for ventilation; in other words to drain the fluid. In reality, it depends on the season. We often try to get to spring, when many children self-resolve their issues as cold season dies down. Infections persisting through spring will often prompt a referral. We tend to be more aggressive in children with developmental delays, or anatomic issues such as having a cleft palate.

Any child who has delayed language skills should have a hearing test. It is so easy to do, and certainly not something we want to miss. It is surprising how many children have mild to moderate amounts of hearing loss detected on routine testing. These are not always enough to treat, but certainly are useful to know about for school purposes.

Speaking of which, we have yet to develop a test for a poor listener. Nor can I fix that one!

d. Better to see you with

When it comes to the eyes, it is vision that matters. Of all the issues that can arise, if you keep this in mind, you will be on the right track. If a condition potentially affects the vision, it is important and potentially urgent; if it doesn't, not so much.

The first potential issue begins at birth. Doctors will look for the *red reflex* in a newborn. This is like the red eye that you will see in a flash photograph. If you notice that only one pupil is red when you take a picture, something is wrong with the other eye. There may be a cataract in the lens that is preventing light to get to the back of the eye. Early identification and treatment can save the vision in that eye. Vision can be permanently lost because the infant brain tends to shut down the nerve inputs that are not being used. If one eye is not sending messages back, the brain will deactivate that nerve. After several months, blindness in that eye is the result, even if the cataract is removed later on.

One of the earliest pleasures for a parent is to know that your child is looking at you. Contrary to what many people believe, babies can see from birth.. Early vision is only a couple of feet away. By 2 months of age, your baby should be able to follow your face across a full 180-degree arc. My youngest, Christopher, was one that didn't. I started getting concerned as the two-month mark approached. Of course, I did not say anything to Sandee, because it was not yet time for alarm. The night before 8 weeks of age, she asked if I had noticed that he was not following. She does not like when I blow off her concerns, but she likes it much less when I validate them. We are lucky to be friends with Dr. Lois Townshend, an excellent pediatric ophthalmologist, who squeezed us in the next day. Christopher passed his exam in the morning, and by the afternoon he was obviously following us. We think that being the third child, he just wanted to make sure we were paying him enough attention.

Newborn eyes normally cross from time to time. This should stop by four months of age. After that, crossing eyes should see the eye doctor. An eye that crosses occasionally is less of a concern than one that is not aligned all the time. Eyes that are not aligned send blurry messages back to the brain. The brain does not like blurring, and once again, may shut down the *lazy* eye's vision. Glasses and or patching can usually help correct this condition, but the occasional child will require surgery.

Extreme sensitivity to light is an important concern that few people realize. If your toddler screams on a sunny day and has to wear sunglasses, this may be a sign of raised pressure in the eye from glaucoma. You may also rarely notice the eyeballs looking waterlogged. Once again, the eye doctor should be involved. Do not be surprised or put off if your primary care provider tries to play down this concern- I learned this 18 years into practice. Call the eye doctor yourself for a pressure check if you must.

Red eyes vary in severity depending on the location of the redness. Most people associate red eyes with conjunctivitis. The conjunctiva is the lining of the eye. Bacterial conjunctivitis is usually goopy, and responds well to antibiotic drops. This prompts me to say that it order to have *junk*-tivitis, you need to have *junk* and –it is, that is, goop. Viral conjunctivitis is usually watery and often goes along with common cold symptoms. Both are very contagious and will lead to prompt exclusion from daycare or preschool. You can also have allergic conjunctivitis, which tends to be itchy. Older kids and

262

adults can describe conjunctivitis as stinging, but it is not truly painful.

Red eyes that are painful can be from more serious causes that should be followed up. Localized redness on the edge of the lash is from a stye, essentially a pimple of the eyelash. These are easily treated with warm soaks and antibiotic ointment. Within a couple of days, they usually pop and drain. Redness on the skin of the lids and around the eye can be from a skin infection, or cellulitis. This is a serious condition. Pain and fever are usually also present. Urgent treatment with antibiotics is needed to prevent a true infection of the orbit, which can spread back into the brain.

Goop in the eyes *without* redness is usually from another cause. The most common reason is a blocked tear duct, which can be explained as follows. The tears drain from the eyes to the nose through little tubes called the tear ducts. These tubes can become clogged. This leads to tear formation while awake, and crusting, sticking together and mild goop after sleeping. Block tear ducts can last for several months after birth. It only requires moist cotton balls to cleanse the eyes, and maybe saline nose drops to loosen any nasal congestion. The only way to fix it permanently is for the eye doctor to insert a probe to open the duct; needless to say, we only recommend this if it has not resolved on its own.

Goopy eyes can also develop in a sinus infection. Think of this like a pipe that has backed up. Sometimes you see the backup in the sink, or in this case, in the eye. The real problem is congestion lower down. This differs from conjunctivitis because there is no redness of the conjunctiva and there are usually cold symptoms present.

We take the eyes for granted until there is a problem. This is human nature. Awareness of the importance of a few simple symptoms, especially pain and impaired vision, will keep him seeing well. That way, the eyes will be more than a window to his soul; they will be his window to the world.

Chapter 11: Joe Safety

a. Keep car seats rear-facing until your baby is 2

Kids and cars have a lot in common. For the early part of their lives, both are expected to run well. In a sense, both are under warranty, because major problems seldom happen. The one major issue not covered by a car warranty is a crash. In the same way, an injury is the most common way that a healthy young person becomes sick. One of the most common places for children to become injured is in the car, and this makes car safety a major priority.

As you know, cars are potentially dangerous due to the speed at which they travel. High speeds translate into high forces. The essence of car safety is reducing the force that the body receives, if a crash should occur. For adults, the main tool is the seat belt. Seat belts work in two ways. First, they prevent us from being ejected from the car. Second, they allow the forces to be distributed across our bones rather than our vital organs. The original lap belt spread the force of a crash across the pelvic bones. Lap/shoulder belts are better because forces are distributed across a much larger area, so that the force in any one spot is reduced. The car seat was invented because seat belts clearly are not appropriate to restrain babies. The seat not only keeps babies from being thrown, it allows forces to be distributed across the plastic and foam rather than the baby.

Car seats should face backwards for as long as possible, at least until the age of 2 years. Most fatal collisions occur when the front of the car crashes into something. When the front of the car crashes, an unrestrained driver or passenger will be thrown forward. Even when restrained, the body's momentum will try to throw it forward. Car seats are not perfect, and if forward facing, babies still have a risk of being propelled forward. On the other hand, a restrained rear facing car seat will typically be stable at the base. The end result is that the top of the car seat will rotate back towards the back seat. This will actually *cocoon* the child under the seat, and if anything, the child will only contact the back seat. For this reason, *children who are rear-facing in the second year of life are four to five times less likely to be killed in a crash*. These numbers speak for themselves.

Parents often express concern about the rear-facing position. A lot of this is parental anxiety from having less ability to visualize the child. While understandable, there are times when we have to override our parental instincts because we know that it is safer for young children to be rear facing. There is also the issue of fit and comfort. Most of our cars have not been designed to fit larger seats rear facing. Toddler legs have a tendency to get scrunched up or go up the back of the seat. In reality, this usually bothers us more than it does them. If a seat really does not seem to fit, most

266

communities have car seat inspectors at the local fire or police station. These technicians have extensive training at making a seat fit as well as possible.

While we are on the subject of seats, I want to put in a plug for maintaining the full toddler car seat for as long as it fits. While many people use 40 pounds as the time to graduate to a booster seat, this is usually too soon. Toddler seats are called *five point seats*, referring to the straps contacting the body on both hips, both shoulders and the chest- in other words, at five points. As we discussed above, more points of contact means spreading out a force over a larger area.

We live in a goal-oriented world. Many of us are motivated by accomplishing a task, and then moving on to the next one. Kids themselves want to be *big*, and as parents, we often encourage this. However, when it comes to safety, using equipment of the proper size is important. Correct fit can make the difference between safe and unsafe, and this is particularly true of car seats.

As my colleague Dr. Paul Schreiber likes to say, you wouldn't put your son in his father's suit, so don't try to put him in his father's seat.

b. Model Safe Behavior

We have all heard the expression, "Do as I say, not as I do." Let's just start by throwing that one away, and replacing it with, "Actions speak louder than words." Although it is more difficult, ultimately our kids' safety depends on the habits that they learn from us. And they learn from us what we show them.

Young children are tremendous learners, much more than what adults realize. They are sponges for knowledge. A large part of what they learn is by observation. This is evident before the first birthday in games like Peek-a-boo. However, their learning is not limited to the times that we are actively teaching. Much of it takes place by simply viewing everyday life.

There is ample evidence that children model their behavior after their parents' behavior. Parents who read to their children have children who read more. Parents who exercise have children who exercise. Parents who smoke are more likely to have children who smoke. While this discussion could have been included in other parts of the book, I chose to put it the section on safety because it may be less obvious that safe parental behavior encourages safe behavior in a child.

Cape Cod has many miles of bicycle trails. It is amazing how often I see young kids riding their bikes with helmets, while the parent rides unprotected without a helmet. First of all, think about who will take care of the children if a parent has a debilitating brain injury. Aside from this, it should not be rocket science to understand that these children will likely *graduate* to abandon their helmets. Believe me when I say that beginning at age of 12 (which is roughly the age of bicycle independence), helmets are unfortunately forsaken by many kids. As with so many things, we eventually emulate our parents, and return to a safe behavior at some point. Our best hope for keeping these kids safe is to be clear about our feelings on safety. The best way to make this statement is through our own safe behaviors.

The same argument can be made for cell phone use in cars, sun protection, and life jackets. Our children will observe our behavior, and probably follow the same pattern as us. Although the results of our actions may not be evident when they are little, this is the ideal time for us to set a good example.

Some of our behaviors translate immediately into increased safety for our children. For example, we know that parents who use seat belts are more likely to use the appropriate car seats for their children. In our relationships, safe behavior not only insulates our children from violence later, it protects them from aggressive behavior as young kids. Perhaps most importantly, avoidance of a gun in the house makes it less likely that our children will be victims of gun violence.

Why do we as parents have trouble grasping the influence of our actions on our children? This is pure speculation, but I am guessing that it is complicated. To begin with, most parents are not psychologists and just may not be aware of how closely they are being watched and imitated. Certain parents will have rose-colored glasses, feeling that they can talk the safety talk, without walking the walk. A few can't see past the parent- child bonding, even if the bonding involves danger. These parents are reluctant to upset their children if they protest. Others are resistant to change, and have difficulty adapting behavior, although it will benefit their children. This is the, "I haven't worn a helmet for 40 years, and nothing has happened to me" group. And some people even have nostalgia for unsafe behavior- "Remember when 10 of us used to ride in the flatbed truck?"

As pediatricians, we encounter all these explanations. Heck, sometimes we even practice them- I have three hockey-playing kids, despite the injuries that occur. One thing I can tell you is that physics does not care about rationalizations that we all make. Injuries happen. Many people do not *get it* until they get it in a way that no one would ever wish upon them; this is, until it happens to their child. You never want to be in that position, especially if your own unsafe behavior may have contributed.

c.   Don't break your brain

My office partner, Dr. Peter Lind, calls me Joe Safety. I mention this as a reflection of the importance I put on child safety. That being said, other safety advocates may strongly disagree with this chapter, because I am speaking more as a practical person than a purist. I think there are limits on how many rules we can ask parents and kids to follow. If we have to make choices, my priority is to protect the brain.

Ninety-nine per cent of the time, pediatricians encourage children and families to be more active. The other one per cent is spent dealing with the injuries that result from being active. There is nothing I like better than to see a school-aged kid with bruises on her shins. I know that sounds strange, but it tells me that she is playing hard. Kids need exercise- it is good for their body, mind and soul. We can't be like the schools that have banned tag for fear that someone will get hurt. What we need to do is reduce the risk of serious injuries. What we need to do is reduce brain injuries.

There are many kids who wear total body armor when learning to ride a bike. That is great, because it protects the child, reassures the parent and possibly removes some of the anxiety around this task. Having said that, many other parents struggle to get their kids to wear any safety gear at all. We can control them when they are young, but it is not long before they are old enough to ride off on their own, and who knows what they are doing once they turn the corner. As a parent, I quickly stopped insisting on kneepads, elbow pads and wrist guards, because it was a losing battle. However, when it comes to their noggins, my kids know that I will enforce helmets to the max.

Any part of the body can be seriously injured- perhaps if I were an elbow or a knee surgeon I would emphasize these parts more- but safety is most importantly about preventing irreparable injuries. In this sense, brain injury wins. The brain is obviously so important to how we function. It controls everything we do, feel and think. More subtle, but equally critical, are the ability to show control over our emotions, and to balance.

The second issue with an injured brain is its reduced capacity to fully repair itself. We used to think of brain injuries in adults as *permanent*, and in young children as less permanent, because a young child's brain was thought to be more *plastic*, or able to adapt. Recent advances in brain science have revealed that both of these concepts are more complicated than previously thought. Still, the bottom line is that of all the organs in the body, the brain is safely the slowest and the worst at repairing itself. As I tell my young patients, if you break your brain, I can't fix it.

The good news is that most brain injuries are preventable. This is another reason to emphasize brain safety. Unintentional brain injuries can be reduced by using car seats, helmets, preventing falls and near-drowning events, and by keeping guns out of the house.

Child abuse prevention is more complicated, but also can be achieved.

For new parents, strap in the car seat when its in use, and when it is out of the car, only put it on the floor in the house (there is less distance to fall.) Constantly supervise your young children, especially around water in the tub or at the beach, and on the playground. When the tricycle or scooter is introduced, make sure a helmet is, too, so that wheels and helmets always go together. Turn in guns to your local police, or at least ensure they are locked in a safe and unloaded.

The only good injury is the one that never happened. This is especially true when it comes to the brain.

d.   What to do if he hits his brain

It happens so fast. One minute he is fine, the next he has fallen and hit his head. There are so many ways it can happen. A baby gate which guarded the stairs was left open or malfunctions, a climber gets up on a table, or you just plain trip with him in your arms. Whatever the cause, you are suddenly in the position of panic and guilt. How do you know what to do? Try to stay calm, and your child will tell you.

Let's start by saying that a good class in first aid can really help you to prepare for these situations. Having said that, it is really difficult to be rational when your own baby is hurt. All that matters is that your most precious possession is hurt. If you can't calm yourself, call for help.

A little bit of a physics refresher can help to guide us on when to worry. As I mentioned elsewhere, the force has a lot to do with the risk and severity of injury. Force is directly related to velocity. This is why high-speed car crashes do more harm than when tripping over a curb. As a parent, you will know that a fall off a balcony, down a flight of stairs, or God forbid, out a window, should worry you more than a roll off the couch. In the Emergency Department, we use this *mechanism of injury* information as well. The risk increases as the force increases.

The other physics principle is that every action has an equal and opposite reaction. That force that the baby brings into the fall is then transmitted to the surface she hits. The surface matters, because a beanbag chair absorbs the force, while concrete reflects it all back to the body. Again, a fall onto a very hard surface increases our concern.

Changes in a child's body are important, too. A baby's skull is made up of several bones that are not fused together yet. This results in soft spots and seams (called sutures) that are ideal for allowing the brain to rapidly grow in the first year. These bones are also softer, which helps with the birth process, but puts the brain and skull at increased the risk of injury. Other worries include the following: babies have big noggins compared to the rest of their bodies, poor head control, limited protective reflexes and a reduced ability to tell us how much is wrong.

That brings us to the important part. How does a child tell us that a head injury is serious? Crying is important, and the message depends on when, and how much. Most children will cry with all but the most trivial injury. If there is no crying and the child goes back about her business- smiling and seemingly unconcerned, then you probably got lucky. Crying will usually stop within a few minutes, depending on the severity of the injury and the pain threshold of the baby. Interestingly, even babies have different pain thresholds (1), although some are too young for you to know yet. Inconsolable crying is a warning sign.

Clearly, loss of consciousness is also a concern. As a parent, this should prompt follow-up. However, do not be surprised if the doctor says everything is all right, because brief loss of consciousness does not always mean a serious injury. But you should let the doctor decide that one. Equally clearly, a child with a persistent loss of consciousness, or one who seems to be becoming more lethargic and less alert needs to be seen immediately. A change in alertness can be a challenge to tell apart from a child who is falling asleep because it is the usual naptime or bedtime. It is very common for children to be tired after a head injury. Again, let the doctor decide if this fatigue is a concern. If he remains unconscious, call 911.

You do *not* have to force your baby to stay awake. Hollywood has this one wrong- there is nothing harmful in itself about falling asleep after you hit your head. The usual chain of events is that there is an injury, followed by a period of crying, followed by fatigue. Many kids fall asleep once the initial event has passed. If in doubt, have the child seen to make sure this is *normal* sleep, but you do not have to keep prodding at them to ward off sleep. A rule of thumb is that a sleeping child after a head blow should wake as he usually does. If you cannot rouse him after sleep, be very concerned.

What about the pupils? Most people will tell me that someone checked the pupils to make sure they were equal. This usually has next to no benefit in an alert child. The size of the pupils is determined the base of the brain, which is also known as the brain stem (assuming there was not a direct blow to the eye itself). The brain stem is also the upper part of the spinal cord. In severe brain injuries, as the brain swells, the pressure can push the brain stem into the base of the skull, leading to a sudden dysfunction of the nerve that controls pupil size, and what doctors call a *fixed, dilated* pupil. As you can imagine, this happens only in the most serious injuries, and usually as the child is becoming comatose. If a pupil is dilated, there are usually a lot of other signs that a major problem exists, namely, an unresponsive child.

276

Vomiting is common after a brain injury. Persistent vomiting is a warning sign. In older kids, we generally allow one or two episodes, if everything else is OK. We are more careful with children under a year, who are less able to tell us about headache and other symptoms. Unsteadiness when walking is also a concern- unless she is at the stage of always being unsteady!

I thought it would be useful for you to know what guidelines Emergency Department staff to reassure that risk for a brain injury in young children is low (PECARN). Any of the following would make you NOT low risk:

1. Suspicion of child abuse
2. Any specific sign of brain injury (trouble moving or seeing etc.)
3. Skull fracture
4. Lethargy on arrival to ER
5. Bulging soft spot
6. Persistent vomiting
7. Seizure
8. Loss of consciousness for more than a few seconds

You do not need to be a doctor, and should not be a doctor for your own child. However, if he is vomiting, lethargic or does anything else that concerns you, get him checked out.

If nothing else, it will help your guilt.

e. Having a gun in your house increases the risk of your child getting shot.

I thought long and hard before writing this chapter, knowing it would upset some people. In the end, I feel it has to be said.

The United States is a great country. We do many great things. We also kill each other with guns at a rate that is much higher than any other high-income country in the world. Adults kill adults. Adults kill children. Children kill children. Adults and children kill themselves. Some are intentional and many are accidental. Even among 5 to 14 year olds, our firearm death rates are 10 times higher than other countries. It has to change.

Some people own guns for hunting; others own them for self-protection. Ironically, research has shown that the presence of a gun in a home increases the rate of homicide and suicide. Gun ownership also makes a person four times more likely to be shot in an assault. In other words, gun ownership does not protect most people.

"Do you have any guns in your house?" This is a simple question, but one that many of us would not think to ask, or would avoid asking. Consider that over one quarter of gun owners with children under age twelve report leaving their guns loaded. The American Academy of Pediatrics considers this an important enough question, that it recently promoted, "National Ask Day."

If you own a gun, do you truly need it? If you are a police officer, the answer will be, "Yes." Do you need to store it at home? The answer is probably, "No." If you insist on having it at home, gun safes are essential. So is the storage of guns unloaded, with ammunition stored in a separate location.

I would urge everyone to watch a recent *20/20* special on how children behave around guns. While it may shock you, it may help you to make a life-saving decision.

f. You childproof. They figure out what you miss.

A nine month old loves to crawl towards the staircase. A ten month old looks first to see if you're paying attention, then crawls for the stairs. And so, two of the most underrated signs of a child's intelligence are demonstrated: the ability to get yourself in trouble, and the ability to manipulate your parents.

My brother, Steve, is not a medical person; he's an engineer. However, he is the father of three boys. He gets credit for the all-time best piece of child safety advice: "The only real childproofing is direct supervision." It has been many years since he said this, but it is still true. I have shared this experience with many patients, and each time I get a kick out of knowing that this was not learned in a classroom or a hospital, but rather, in the parenting trenches.

Life is an adventure for a child. They are looking to explore and learn. However, most kids do not understand the potential dangers that stand in their way. Each child explores differently, and some styles are definitely more danger-prone than others. There are the human wrecking balls. There are climbers and jumpers. There are mouthers. There are runners. There are daredevils. You will learn why some families lay all the kitchen chairs down on the floor, while others need harnesses to keep the kids close. And you will learn how to become suspicious when it is *too* quiet.

Child safety devices are invaluable, but only as a means to slow down Miss Trouble. Every lock can be picked. Every gate can be climbed. Every outlet device can be pulled. They delay, but do not prevent problems. You can improve your safety odds by having a room where everything that is potentially dangerous has been removed. If you don't have an entire room, a playpen or gated area can work as well. Watch out for the toys of older siblings, which are often choking hazards. You can tell an older sibling that he is in charge of making sure you don't leave any small objects on the ground; this will help her watch out for herself, too.

You may have to get creative with other techniques to improve your safety. Our third child, Christopher, was the climber. He could scale a table or piece of furniture in a blink. Prior to his second birthday, we taught him the word *cannonball*. Recognizing that he was going to climb no matter what we did, we taught him to announce his jumps with this word. Three syllables take a while to say when you're 2, and it bought just enough time for us to turn around with outstretched arms.

Multitasking while watching the children can be potentially dangerous. All parents of more than one child multitask, by definition. Still, it is important to realize that our brains do not truly do two things at once. Sophisticated research shows that when attempting to multitask, our brains quickly *ping-pong* from one activity to the next; for example, from watching the baby to getting dressed to watching the baby etc. This ping-pong effect is too fast for us to notice consciously. Electronics are a major source of distraction, and the advent of smart phones has brought this issue to a new level. It even has a name- *texting while parenting*. Some researchers believe too much focus on our devices has led to a recent increase in child injuries.

There are few sounds worse than the cry of pain. We have all heard that sound, and it can come from out of nowhere. Closely supervising your children will help to spare them from that terrible sound, and the consequences of the injury which caused it.

Chapter 12: Random Stuff

a.   Second child guilt

You have just delivered your second child. What you may not have expected while you were expecting is a whole new kind of guilt. Essentially, you feel, "I can't do for the first one what I used to be able to do for the first one, and I can't do for this one what I used to do for the first one." This feeling is almost universal for second-time mothers. I call it *second child guilt*.

In fact, this feeling may well have begun earlier in the pregnancy. This is especially true if you had any health issues that required you to go on bed rest. Even if you were healthy, your energy and your ability to run around certainly will have gone down. Your partner or relative may have had to take over some of your duties, be they dinner, bath or bedtime.

Feelings intensify when you leave for the hospital, in particular if your older child is a toddler, and has had limited experience away from you at bedtime. Sometimes there are tantrums, just to twist the knife, and other times relatives are a little too honest about the first night without you. Speaking on the phone has a tendency to backfire; your intentions are good, but the sound of your voice (or sight of you on *Skype* or *Facetime*) may well propel a child who was coping into one who is upset.

Your time at the hospital with Number Two is just as precious as it was with Number One. In some ways, this time is even more precious, because you will not have the same one-on-one capability at home that you had the first time. The newborn hospital stay gives you a brief opportunity to stare and cuddle, with no laundry, groceries, work or other distractions. Take full advantage of it. In fact, you may enjoy it more than the first time, because you will be much more calm about the whole prospect of what is involved in raising a baby.

When you get home, you will almost certainly have less time than you did with the first. You may find yourself amazed that you thought that looking after one child was busy. It was, but everything is relative. You will probably find that the new baby book is largely left incomplete. With a first child, you might have had the chance to talk with other first time parents that you meet at a coffee shop or restaurant. It is like being part of a club, and there is instant bonding with other new members. With a second child, you do not want to bond- you need to get in and out of the grocery store, so that you aren't late for preschool pick-up. You have come to truly appreciate drive-thrus, and may be contemplating home delivery!

When you get home, you can anticipate some degree of backlash from Number One. This may take the form of attention seeking, crying or a regression in behavior. It is usually not as bad as most parents fear, although I have known older siblings to ask if the baby could be put out with the trash! You just need to keep reminding yourself that you are giving your child a playmate, which will become worth its weight in gold. You are also teaching Number One the very important lesson that, although he is the center of the universe, there are a few other stars out there, too. To be honest, I am often pleasantly surprised by how well older siblings do when a new baby arrives. One of the most common problems is that a preschool age sister wants to be a second mother, and tries to do more than what is safe. The range of reactions varies; do not be surprised or disappointed if a sibling does not seem that interested in a new baby. This is also perfectly normal.

Siblings older than 5, sometimes have a harder time than younger children. These kids have been only children for much longer, and are old enough to achieve more secondary gain from misbehaving. It is a big adjustment to have a baby become the new center of attention. Including an older child in prenatal events can go a long way to make for a good adjustment, as can repeated reminders of the *hero* status that a younger child will confer upon a significantly older sibling. Many years later, you can still remind the oldest of the smiles that the baby gave him. This can come in handy when the baby wants to hang out with older child's friends.

Oh, and a little bribery never hurts. A gift *from the newborn* to an older sibling of any age can assist the bonding process.

b. With two children you can play man on man defense; with three you have to play a zone

My pediatrician friend, Michael Peer, told me that one of the fathers in his practice came up with this great expression. If you are not a basketball fan, let me put it this way: you are out-numbered. You will find yourself saying, "I have her, you have him...that one is okay for a minute."

There is no question that adding more children adds more work-more bedtimes, more pick-ups and drop-offs, more illnesses, and potentially more fighting. Each consecutive child adds an element to the equation, but the consensus among parents seems to be that the largest increase in work (barring multiple births) is going from the second to the third child. There is something about this point that increases the chaos in your life. This is especially true if the kids come in quick succession. Looking back on this time, many mothers feel like there are about five years that are a blur.

Having three children gets a bad rap because of the fear that it is *always two against one* or that there will be a middle child syndrome. The truth is much more involved. If you simply look at gender and birth order, there are eight different possibilities: girl-girl-girl, girl-girl-boy etc. When you add in the variations in spacing between children, and the differences in the their personalities, there are many combinations of experiences that a family can have. I am no expert on birth order and personality, but in real life, it is safe to say certain birth positions allow certain personality traits more opportunity. For example, an oldest sister can be nurturing to her younger siblings, and a youngest child is more prone to being over-protected.

How many children are right for you? This is no easy question. It depends on your health, relationship, financial situation, religion and most of all, on your personality. Most of us have a sense of how many we want early on, but it is wise to reassess as you go. Many people are surprised by the chaos that comes with multiple children. It is very difficult to have eight children when you have a need for control in your life. Issues with your current children can also make it challenging to think about having more. It makes sense to let your personalities determine a maximum ideal number, and then your circumstances determine if you need to reduce it.

No matter how many children you have, you will almost certainly be struck by how each one is different. It really is remarkable the number of different ways that genes can combine. And you will almost certainly feel like you cannot imagine life without any of them.

c. Good foster and adoptive parents have a special place in heaven; bad ones have a special place in hell

In a future life, I would like to reform the care of children whose parents are incapable of caring for them. On the whole, this is one of the most difficult aspects of providing child health care. We have talked about the biologic parents elsewhere, but I would like to consider the state of foster and adoptive care, and of the people involved in it.

For starters, it needs to be said that social services/child welfare has to be one of the most difficult and stressful fields in which a person could work. These people are making extremely important decisions about where and with whom a child will live. They face incredible amounts of anger and upset. They do not always have all the important information. They are underfunded, overworked and underpaid, often inexperienced, and the laws of their jurisdiction limit their decisions. Under these circumstances, it is no surprise that the system is broken.

One of the major problems with foster care is the shortage of good, capable foster parents. As a pediatrician, you see all types of surrogate caregivers. Unfortunately, most are less than ideal. From the child's perspective, if a parent is unable to participate, the next best alternative would be to have a stable, caring, capable and consistent home in which a child can be raised. This will minimize the loss that the child experiences. What we see, more often than not, is that children go back and forth, from home to home, and in and out of parental custody.

I have always thought that when there is a divorce, the kids should get the house, and the parents should have to come and go. It is too bad that the same principle doesn't apply to foster care. Of course, this is unrealistic, but it often seems that the child's interests stop being served once they are in *the system*. How many of us, as adults, could function well within the uncertainty of multiple transitions, and unknown caregivers?

Most commonly, a child will go into the care of a relative. In the right circumstances, this can be terrific. If a family member is willing and able, there is a sense of continuity, and the child will feel like he belongs. There may already be a relationship with the caregiver and with cousins. However, sometimes the issues that plague the parent(s) originated in the grandparents house. Other times, grandparents (or great grandparents) are just getting too old to be able to meet the demands of young. There are many grandparents in my practice who have assumed the primary caregiver role. Most of them should get a free pass into heaven. It is not unusual for the grandparents to be raising the children of their adopted foster children, who just were not able to make it themselves as parents. These grandparents almost always look tired. The care needs often exceed those of other children. At some point, they often have to refuse to take on a third or fourth grandchild because the stress on their health is so great. Despite their incredible past commitment, they can be left with a feeling of overwhelming guilt. This seems so unfair.

Unrelated foster parents are a mixed bag. Some are fantastic, having chosen foster care as a career, often a second career. It is fairly easy to pick these people out when you meet them. I have one extremely spry seventy-five-year old who comes into the office with one baby in a backpack, and a second in a front pack. She is a specialist in temporary custody of babies. How fortunate are the babies who get to be nurtured by her at least for a while, at this critical time of development. It is amazing to watch a neglected infant gain milestones in leaps and bounds when given the chance.

On the other hand, some people seem more concerned with the money received for taking on a foster child than with the child. Rumors of abuse within the homes of foster care providers are not uncommon, but as is usually the case, the evidence required to remove children from these providers is lacking. There are several children I have seen grow up in long term foster care who just did not get what they deserved.

To make matters worse, parents often float in and out of the child's life, in an attempt to reunite a family. For every success story, there are multiple failures. The result is that the child ends up further scarred, both by the neglect in the parent's home, and by the re-traumatization that occurs with the re-separation. It is always a shame to see a child who starts to thrive in a foster or pre-adoptive home, then end up a mess again when he is returned to his birth home. Parents should have to do a better job at proving their recovery prior to be being given a second, third or fourth chance.

What does all this have to do with you as a new parent? Fair question. For starters, it serves to emphasize the challenges of parenthood for all of us. It also makes me feel lucky to have been raised by good and loving parents. Finally, I do think it is just worth being aware of the struggle that some children endure on a daily basis, and what we, as a society, should be doing to help.

If you or someone you know has what it takes to be a good foster parent, the world could really use you.

d. Dealing with a rare diagnosis

Uncharted waters. That is where you may have found yourself. Rough, scary uncharted waters. How do you stay afloat if your child has been diagnosed with an uncommon, serious medical condition?

We take good health for granted. Part of the assumption of good health is that our children will be born healthy. In fact, an enormous number of steps must occur correctly for a healthy baby to result. There are so many steps that most of us would rather not think about it. Unless, of course, we had no choice.

Each of the steps in the normal function of a human being has the possibility of going wrong. In fact, each step does go wrong on very rare occasion. As a result, a vast number of conditions exist where one error occurred in development, or one chemical reaction does not happen correctly. Most times this occurs due to one error in the child's genetic makeup. It can be as simple as one protein that is not produced properly, or a small missing or extra piece of genetic material.

Many of the conditions that result from these errors of development occur in only one in a million children. Sometimes there are less than one hundred other children affected in the entire world. News that your child is affected is shocking, and life changing. There is usually very little time to adapt because your baby may be very sick, or have significant special needs. It is difficult to know where to turn.

Each condition has its own set of symptoms and needs. It is still worth looking at them as a group because there are many common strategies to help parents. If your child has a rare condition, chances are you have ended up in a dedicated children's hospital. The team at the hospital will become your child's lifeline, and yours, as well. Your specialist(s) and specialty team will teach you about the condition. This will help you to understand what to expect in the months and years ahead.

Each diagnosis has its own set of problems. Consider a more common condition, such as Down Syndrome, to illustrate the point. All children with Down Syndrome have similarities in their facial appearance. You may not know that having a lazy eye, recurrent ear infections, hole in the heart, bowel obstruction and a long list of other afflictions affect some but not all children with Downs. The extent of these associated problems often has a large impact on the quality of life

In a similar way, your child's rare condition will have its own set of issues. Since the diagnosis is rare, the issues may not always be as well understood as in Down Syndrome. However, generally, your child's condition will have a core set of features, which all affected children share, and others that are present only in some children. Your specialty team will perform tests to investigate which your child's individual issues.

Once the initial testing is completed, the team will educate you about your child's problems. Some children will have delays in development and seizures, In this case, you will learn to recognize and respond to seizures, to administer medication, and to look for side effects. Others will have problems with feeding. It may be necessary to uses a specialized tube to administer feedings, and you will become familiar with specialized formulas or feeding systems.

Metabolic disorder is the term for a huge group of rare illnesses where the body has a problem with making or breaking down a protein, sugar or other essential chemical. Each metabolic problem has its own consequences. Problems with normal metabolism can commonly cause low blood sugar or acid buildup. Too much of a certain chemical can also build up in organs such as the liver, brain or heart, which can make them malfunction. You will need to be taught your child's potential for emergency problems, and signs when emergency care is required.

Needless to say, this all can be completely overwhelming. It is clear why your specialty team is so important to your child and to you. You will lean on them heavily for information and support. Support of other families who have a child with the same condition can be a huge help. Families with a new diagnosis can be helped by those with more experience. The Internet makes this help much more readily available, especially when only one hundred children in the world share the same problem. Families from Alaska to New Zealand can now communicate, connect and share information. Try to limit your communicating to people and subjects that will help you and your child. Remember that even with rare conditions, the Internet also has the potential to be a soapbox for those who love to complain.

Remember that your child also remains an individual. All kids are different, whether they share blonde hair, asthma, ADD or a rare diagnosis. As a parent, you will become the world's expert on your own child. You will know his every move, and interpret things that are lost on others. You will also read about the body, possibly developing a fund of knowledge on a subject in which you previously knew nothing. You will perform duties that you never considered or of which you never felt capable. You will have no choice.

And you will advocate. Your child will need you even more than most others. You will likely need to be a *squeaky wheel*, at times when needs are not being met, or the team is pushing too hard. And you will have to care for yourself, because you and your family will be the main caregivers for your child. There will be adjustments in family dynamics, and these will not be easy. Everything will have to be adjusted.

You will also educate others, including your extended family, neighbors and friends. You may be surprised to learn that your health care providers have never heard of your child's diagnosis. This is not as terrible as it sounds at first. There are so many conditions that no one can know them all. However, they will have cared for other rare conditions. Good providers will educate themselves, but also will listen to you. If you have a strong relationship, you will listen to the tips that their general medical and nursing experience with special needs children has taught them.

Finally, a practical point. Get a letter from your specialist (or an involved primary care provider), which outlines the diagnosis, the problems, and any steps which need to be taken in case of specific emergencies. Keep this with you at all times. Unfortunately, some providers, especially those with whom you do not have a pre-existing relationship, do not always listen to parents. In an emergency, presenting a letter from another professional can avoid delays, errors and serious consequences.

Because when it comes to rare diagnoses, doctor does not always know best. That does not stop us from acting as if we do.

e. Beware of the electronic babysitter

It used to be that pediatricians worried about children who were spending more time watching television than engaging in interactive play. We used to promote campaigns like 'Screen Free Week", to make the point. With the advent of mobile devices, this has been elevated to an entirely new level. In the right hands, and with the wrong supervision, the opportunity exists for children to spend a large percentage of their waking hours viewing a screen.

Many businesses have long had televisions in their waiting rooms. Pediatricians' offices were unlikely to be among those who did, because we know that too many children watch too much television. It would be hypocritical of us to say one thing, and do another, just as much as if we rode bikes without wearing helmets. When the time came for us to embrace Wi-Fi for the office, I similarly kept it password-protected so that kids were not surfing while waiting. A couple of years ago, portable DVD players started to accompany some kids while they waited. Smart phones and data plans now make it absolutely commonplace for kids to be viewing something when I enter an exam room.

To be fair, most parents instruct their kids to turn off when the visit begins. I certainly have been known to keep people waiting, and cannot blame anyone who is trying to stay occupied during this time. There can also be many fewer interruptions from a sibling who is gaming than from one who has to sit quietly during a visit. And I admit to being impressed by a two-year-old who has better command of an iPhone than me, although that is really not saying too much.

Call me old-fashioned, but I love to see a mother reading an actual book with pictures to her son. And I am always impressed by a family who has used the table paper creatively - a nice drawing, a game of X's and O's or Hangman. Is this just a sign of my age, or is there something to the intuition that people interact more and better when electronics are not involved?

I have spoken previously about the need to speak to children to promote language development. Here my focus is different- what is the impact of spending too much *time* plugged in, even if you are comfortable that the content of the electronics is not in itself harmful? In other words, how do benign video games and electronics affect children, by virtue of the time spent, and the absence of the time spent doing other activities?

The short answer is we do not know. In reality, the computer revolution is occurring so quickly that by the time researchers look at a subject, the device being used may already be out of date. Having said that, there are several areas that are important to consider, and in which data will undoubtedly be gathered in the next decade.

Social development is extremely important for babies. We know, for example, that play between parents and children helps to build strong connections. Imaginative play helps to build creativity and resilience. Studies of socially deprived children, most notably, those who were adopted from institutions, tells us that early deprivation has permanent effects on IQ, recognition of faces and other social behaviors, and emotional health. Is screen time a milder form of social deprivation?

There is very little research available on the social development of children with increased screen time. We do know that even background television reduces the amount and quality of verbal interactions between children and adults. So, it is very likely that a screen in the child's *foreground* would do the same. Face to face time is almost certainly going to be lower, if my observations of toddlers watching screens are correct. Previous research on television viewing has suggested that quality matters, in addition to quantity.

For example, deliberate attempts to educate a child with electronics do not seem to affect play time spent with the child, while viewing that is purely for entertainment may reduce play time. Simply put, it suggests that using the television as a babysitter, at the expense of interactive time, is not a good idea. The same could be expected of a smart phone or tablet.

Areas of behavior which can be easily measured, have also been easier to study when it comes to electronics. For example, attention span has been measured in kids with higher screen time. Although not definitive, the early suggestion is that electronics can promote lower attention span in children at risk. The theory is that video stimuli change rapidly, and condition the child to only having to focus briefly.

Physical health changes are clearer. The risk of obesity increases in older children with greater screen time. This is likely a combination of eating while viewing, slowing of the rate of metabolism, and the fact that physical activity is not taking place. New data suggests that high blood pressure is also more common with increasing screen time.

Much more information is on the horizon, as electronics become a fixture in our world. For this generation of children, we have to make decisions with less information than we would like. I think the important thing is to be aware that risks potentially exist, and that it is just as important as ever to spend face-to-face time with our kids.

Over 600 years ago, Chaucer first observed that "mighty oaks from tiny acorns grow." (1) While he had no knowledge brain biology, we now know that the quality of the *oak* is based how the nerves grow, connect and are pruned. As parents, we are the gardeners, and need to give those oaks a chance to grow well by spending time and energy. You still get out of it what you put into it.

f. Be an informed media consumer- and teach your children, too

Do you remember the ads between the cartoons you watched as a kid? The ones with the amazing toys. Did you ever actually get one and then experience how poorly it worked in real life? This sums up my view of advertising. The job of most companies is to sell and advertising makes this process easier. Although some products and some media are fantastic, most are not. Teaching your child from an early age to be an informed media consumer will reap many rewards.

Beginning when my kids were little, I used to question their cartoon ads. "Why do you think they advertise toys and sugar cereals during shows that you guys watch?" I knew my point had been made when they started to chime in, "So you'll buy stuff", before the words were not even out of my mouth. It is never too early for children to become media savvy.

If you think this is overly cynical, consider discount baby socks that have *golden arches*, or *Crayola* logos. Even diapers that display Elmo are there for a reason, as much as I love Elmo. Children are being branded from a very early age. You can test this yourself- two year-olds will be able to recognize the logo of whatever stores you frequent regularly, just like they can find their own cereal in the cupboard.

There are two basic parts of media awareness. The first part is just the basic knowledge of the *extent* to which advertisers attempt to manipulate our actions. Advertising is everywhere in our society. While some advertising is obvious, we now live in an age where our Internet use patterns will be monitored, and where our online views have been personalized. Even young children will be affected, because they are exposed to the advertising that accompanies the media. Parents are being targeted if you click on links for children's products. As a quick experiment, I interrupted my writing of this chapter and logged on to the PBSkids.org website, which is undoubtedly the highest quality and most educational of American children's television. The first thing I noticed is a links for their shows. The parent's link brings you to an option to *shop PBS*. I wonder how long it will be before my search engine home page would start to reflect children's toy advertising.

The second part of media awareness involves knowledge of the effects that the *content* of media has on all of us, but especially children. This is incredibly important, and almost certainly undervalued by mainstream society. There is now a huge body of evidence to show that children are affected when they view media. This includes influences on aggressive behavior, risky sexual behavior, substance use, and disordered eating. (1) While we might think of these as being issues for older children and adults, the seeds of what we consider normal are planted in our young children. For example, few would be surprised to hear that a child living in a violent household might act out violently. We need to be aware that the media that enters our house is influencing behavior as well.

I used to be a skeptic of this, having grown up watching anvils drop on *Wile E Coyote, Godzilla* destroying Japan, not to mention my share of heavyweight title fights. After all, I became a pediatrician. The part that is missing from this equation is that I am not a person prone to violence, and grew up in a loving household. In children who are prone to violence, aggressive media promote this violent tendency. In other words, allowing your aggressive child to watch *World Wrestling Entertainment* is asking for him to become more aggressive.

Even for those of us who are *normal* (whatever that is), watching violent behavior (or casual unprotected sexual behavior, or smoking, or depictions of only women who are skinny) influences

301

our thinking as to what constitutes normal. In other words, if we are inundated by images of drug use, violence or chemically and surgically altered bodies, we start to slowly be influenced unconsciously and consciously about what is normal. This is extremely important for developing minds. If you are skeptical, think about the acceptability in normal language of words that would have resulted in a bar of soap to the mouth for previous generations.

It has been fifty years since Marshal McLuhan coined the phrase, "The medium is the message "(2). How true it has become that media now dictates normal behavior to society. It is critically important for us to be aware of these effects, not just for our children, but also for ourselves. To benefit from modern technology, we have to control it, not the other way around.

Chapter 13: No Excuse for Abuse

a. If I smell cigarettes, your child is exposed to second hand smoke.

Experience has taught me patience. I once suggested to the father of an asthmatic that he quit smoking. He told me that he was six months in drug recovery and did not want to push it. I congratulated him and replied that he should take his time with the smoking. In other words, people's lives are more complicated than they might appear. Still, rose-colored glasses can sometimes affect our vision as much as cigarette smoke.

People are smoking less than in the past, at least in most areas. Parents who smoke are generally doing better at avoiding places where their children will be directly exposed. But there is a lot more work to be done. The smell of cigarettes is too common in doctors' exam rooms. Most of these people swear that they smoke outside. But if I can smell it, it's a sure thing that Junior is breathing it, especially if she is an infant that is frequently being held.

I try every means possible to get parents to reduce their children's smoke exposure *while they are working on quitting*. Smoking in a different room does not count. If you are cooking in one room, the smell of food is in the whole house. Smoking with the window open is not much better; neither is smoking in the basement. Smoking outside with a jacket that is taken off before coming back inside is probably better, as is changing when you get home from work, although if I can still smell smoke in the office, I do wonder how well the parent is doing at home.

As for electronic cigarettes, there is only very limited research. E-cigarettes are basically nicotine that is vaporized in water. They do eliminate many of the other chemicals that are in traditional tobacco cigarettes. Even so, it is too early to know their exact risk, and whether they are a potential tool to be used while quitting altogether (2).

There are many tools available to help a smoker quit. These are beyond the scope of this book. I would like to mention one concept that doctors use, which is really important and useful when you are approaching quitting. It is called the *stages of change* approach. It describes the steps that a person's mind goes through while quitting. Briefly, it begins with the *contemplation* of quitting. You are thinking about it. From there it moves to *preparation* and *action*. Just as important, are *maintenance* and *relapse*, picking yourself up, and circling back to preparation and action again.

Using this approach can be invaluable in the ongoing struggle to quit and to stay quit. More than anything, it gives you a mental framework, and it helps to label where you are at currently. It also helps you realize that relapse is to be expected for many people, and that there is a way to get back to a better place.

If you are a smoker, think about in which stage you currently reside. Maybe this discussion will have you considering a move one step forward. You will never have a better reason than your child's health.

In the meantime, cutting back helps, too.

b. Parenting under the influence

You might me surprised to learn that pediatricians are often experts in substance abuse. I am probably more surprised than you that it has worked out that way for me. I have seen the damage done by the needle, the pills, the powder, the weed, and the bottle.

Addiction is a scourge. Intoxication is highly overrated. Both can destroy relationships and ruin families. You know this, too. Possibly you have seen it. What you may not have seen is the way that substance abuse plays out repetitively in families like the same bad movie.

We have already discussed the physical effects of a mother's drug use on an unborn baby, and the withdrawal that can occur once the infant is born. It is worth repeating that watching a newborn withdraw is a terrible sight. Unfortunately, the number of withdrawing babies tripled between 2000 and 2010, and who knows where it will go from there. Cigarette smoking can add to a newborn's withdrawal, as well as increasing the baby's chances of being born at low birth weight. Smoking also increases the baby's risk for Sudden Infant Death Syndrome, among other problems. Alcohol use causes Fetal Alcohol Syndrome, a leading cause of intellectual impairment.

Drug users often have other medical baggage. Many addicted mothers expose their babies to the Hepatitis C virus, which is a leading cause of liver cancer in young adulthood. There is currently no treatment which can be taken during pregnancy to prevent this transmission. HIV is the most serious infectious risk to a baby, but syphilis and other sexually transmitted infections, and tuberculosis are all more common in addicts.

Society seldom thinks of the addicted mother's struggles during and after pregnancy. Many would argue that this is justified because of the harm she has done to her baby. To be honest, I have mixed feelings about it. There is no question that addiction is powerful. I never met an addict who planned to end up that way. Pregnancy among active addicts is seldom planned. Life situations can be determined by poor upbringings or poor decisions at a young age, although addiction crosses all societal boundaries. Having said that, there is no excuse for remaining addicted while pregnant or once you are a parent. Treatment programs are readily available these days. When addicts are using, they are weaker than their problem(s).

The emotional effects of having a child while addicted are torturous on those parents who care, which is the vast majority that I see. To begin, there is a constant sensation of being judged, which is valid, because mothers in this situation are constantly evaluated to see how they are doing with their babies. Evaluating a parent-addict is essential to see if there is any hope of bringing the child home. The state Department of Social Services (or whichever name it goes by) will be informed and make a decision as to what will become of the child at the time of discharge. Many possible decisions can occur, depending on whether the addiction was in the past or present, how compliant the mother has been with treatment and her medical visits, and whether there is a strong family support network. Social Services can do everything from sending the baby home with the parent to mandating treatment to removing the child from the parent(s) care.

Guilt is a very common emotion among addicted mothers, although it is rarely expressed. There is the guilt of being addicted, the guilt of passing on infectious diseases, and the guilt of not being able to adequately provide for the child. I am not making a judgment about this, merely an observation. The guilt can be expressed as fear- for example, a fear of passing on HIV. It can also clearly be a fear of losing the child's custody. Anger is also commonly seen. Sometimes this is just a mother's unwillingness to confront her own issues, or be honest with herself. Other times it is anger at being treated as a second-class citizen, which some health care workers make no bones about doing. Sometimes guilt comes out as a need to overachieve- to be a *supermom* to make up for the addiction.

The emotional effects on a child can be far worse than the parent experiences. Most times the child goes into foster care. As we discuss elsewhere, good foster situations are less common than bad ones. Many children bounce from home to home. They are unable to form strong attachments at this most critical time in their emotional development. Extended families not uncommonly take temporary care of a child. Grandparents are frequently thrust into parental roles. The results of this can range from life saving to a repetition of the dysfunction that led to the mother's difficulties in the first place. The boom of drug-addicted babies has not been accompanied by a similar growth in the resources of Social Services. Caseworkers are over-worked and underpaid. Mistakes inevitably occur. Babies have ended up in situations where their wellbeing is at risk.

One of the hardest situations we encounter is the addicted parent who comes in and out of the life of her child. The intentions are usually good. The results can be disastrous. In the early months, an intermittent visitor can be fine, as long as she is not disruptive to the baby's care. It becomes much more difficult once the child is old enough to understand that Mommy is not there. Imagine a long, drawn-out breakup, where there are brief periods of reunion, followed by further disappointment and sadness. My sister-in-law Julie calls this killing someone by breaking one bone at a time. Sometimes it is better to just get it over with.

When a non-reformed addict has custody of her child, terrible things can happen. The consequences can range from malnutrition to sexual abuse to unintentional injury. Physical neglect or abuse is relatively easy to detect, provided the child is brought in for care. Emotional neglect can be harder to determine, at least initially. Many, many times the pediatrician's office offers a frustratingly vivid view of the difficulties. You know that the home is not happy. You see dysfunction play out, even during doctor's visits, but you do not have enough evidence to file a report with Social Services. Our instincts are to scoop up the child and look after him ourselves. Instead, we look for and ask about ways in which we might help. We get the community involved, whether it is the visiting nurse, substance abuse program, or another local agency. These people become our eyes and ears away from the office. If in doubt, we file a report, but most are *screened out;* in other words, no case is opened.

Most of the issues we have discussed above can be applied to fathers, too. Sadly, most fathers in these situations are nowhere to be found, or it would be better if they were out of the picture. I have joked that I no longer know how to make rounds on the baby of a happy, invested couple with no major psychosocial issues. It seems to be a small minority of families anymore. Sarcasm aside, it is still a joy to welcome a baby into a happy family.

Violence is a common companion of substance abuse. This is especially true when intoxication is active. The safety of a mother is crucial for her to be able to function well in her new role. All too often, we have to involve the hospital's security staff, and occasionally the police, to keep a dangerous man off the maternity ward. We try hard to ensure that violent fathers do not have access to children and their mothers after discharge.

Although this chapter is largely unhappy, I have to take a moment to celebrate the people who have overcome addiction for the sake of their families, and who have done a great job as parents. I can't mention you by name, but several of your faces are firmly in my head while writing these words. You are truly my heroes.

Our society faces many, many problems. There is no one simple fix. But if I could do only one thing, I would get rid of drugs and alcohol.

c.   Talk to your doctor about sexual and relationship abuse

Doctors pride themselves on their ability to make the right diagnosis. When it comes to detecting abuse, most of us are downright awful. For this, we need your help.

Child abuse is shockingly common. It is estimated that up to one in four children is the victim of some type of abuse (1). This does not include verbal abuse, or being the witness to abuse of a parent by a significant other. All of these conditions have serious adverse effects on a child's well being. Children who are abused or witnesses to abuse have a vastly increased risk of medical problems, emotional problems and relationship problems (2). This makes the prevention and early detection of child abuse critically important. It also makes the doctor's lack of ability to diagnose it all the more tragic.

It is with the best of intentions that physicians miss so much abuse. Without a disclosure from a patient or family member, it is a difficult diagnosis. We are all trained to be wary of certain injury patterns, like burns in the shape of a cigarette, or repeated broken bones. Unfortunately, it is seldom this obvious in primary care. Most single abusive physical injuries closely imitate the regular injuries kids get all the time- bruises and scrapes. A recurring pattern is suspicious, as are more serious injuries, but the main problem for doctors is that we lack sufficient evidence to make a case for abuse, in the same way that police may not be able to gather enough evidence to charge a suspect with another crime.

Sexual abuse is even more elusive. We look for a new onset of urinary accidents, pain with urination and behavior changes. These are by no means specific to abuse. We know that 75 percent of documented sexually abused children have no visible evidence of injury, either because the abuse did not cause an injury, or because it healed without scarring.

We try to interview children on their own as well as with their parents. At a young age, it is very difficult to get children to make a reliable disclosure. Imagine a child of that age talking to a strange adult about anything, let alone abuse. Skilled pediatric nurses and doctors are able to put some kids at ease, and create an environment where a child feels comfortable talking, but this is an uphill battle. Specialized teams and facilities now exist where a child can be interviewed, examined and photographed, if necessary, with law enforcement officials present but concealed. This can benefit the collection of information, preserve evidence and avoid repeated traumatization of a child who has to tell multiple people the same story.

The purpose of this chapter is to encourage you to be vigilant so that abuse may be avoided and so that it can be reported early when it has occurred.

When dating, be aware of people that feel the need to be in control. Be proactive yourself if you are being pressured or abused. It is easy to misjudge a person early in a relationship, but once you realize that a problem exists, try to deal with it early. Have an addicted abuser seek treatment for substance abuse. Recognize that repeated apologies followed by further abuse are a telltale sign that the problem will not go away.

Leaving an abusive relationship is a different road for every victim. While people who have not been through it have trouble understanding why abuse victims stay, a closer look makes the difficulties clear. You need to first realize what is occurring, which can be deceptively hard when you are living it. Then, you have to overcome the legitimate fear of harm occurring after you leave. You need to have a place to go, someone to whom you can turn, enough money and resources to live, and enough courage to face the embarrassment that comes with starting again. If you have children, they can be the source of your courage. They can help you break the cycle.

Sexual abuse has to be destigmatized by all of us. Remember that most abuse perpetrators are people we know. Do not fall into the *Snidely Whiplash syndrome*, named after the villain in the *Dudley Do-right* cartoons. Most abusers do not wear black top hats and capes; nor do they drive white vans. They are most often people that we know and trust; that is, family members and friends. And they are most often men. Be very selective about whom you allow to watch your children. Be wary of behavior changes, especially those with certain sexualized behaviors. Masturbation is normal for young children. Straddling a stuffed animal in a sexual pose is not. If you are not sure, ask your doctor.

313

Many people carry the baggage of some sort of abuse in their own childhood. If this includes you, try to be aware of your own issues and get help before you enter parenthood. If you have yet to do so, the sooner you start, the better. It can make the difference in breaking the cycle for your children.

Chapter 14: What's up with the Doc?

a. God's gifts

From pediatricians to parents:

1. Listening.
2. Treating your child like we would want ours treated.

From parents to pediatricians:

1. Raising nice children.
2. Understanding that listening to another parent may make us late for you.
3. Saying, "Thank you."

From pediatricians to toddlers:

1. The words *no shots today*, *all done* and *bye-bye*.
2. Remembering that they did not cause our bad day.

From toddlers to pediatricians:

1. A smile rather than a scream.
2. Playing peek-a-boo back with us.

b. The list

You know. *That list.* The one with the parents on it who are really…. um, well….neurotic. No, there is no such list. Honest.

Being a parent equals worrying. This is the way we are programmed; the way Mother Nature designs us, so that we will be responsible for our children. Sure, some of us do it more than others, and mothers generally do it more often than fathers. And although too much worry can be counter-productive, my personal opinion is that pediatric caregivers who do not understand that parents worry due to love, need to reevaluate their career choice.

That being said, there are ways that worrying can be channeled, shall we say, more effectively. To begin, remember that pediatricians and their staff care about your child. They want to help. Courtesy and respect will go a long way. Please do not swear at the staff. I know that sounds crazy but it happens. If you have to get angry, get angry with the doctor. Otherwise, you are probably just shooting the messenger. You deserve courtesy in return, and your concerns should be taken seriously. Anger is a last resort- if your concerns are not being heard, then do what you need to do.

Insight is a beautiful thing. I love when people say, "You must think I'm crazy", or "Here she comes again." It shows that you recognize your worrying may not be logical. It also shows that you appreciate having a place to go to be reassured. Since worrying is usually not logical, we get it. You care about your child, and want to make sure he is OK. My job is to help you, and I'm happy to do so.

Listening to the advice you are given also goes a long way. If I tell you that antibiotics won't help, it is because they probably won't help. If you have a strong reason to believe that you are getting incorrect advice, by all means, ask questions, and explain your concerns. As we discussed earlier, sometimes parents do know best. Pushing too hard, too often, can lead many providers to offer treatments that are unnecessary. No one likes conflict, and many providers will offer an unnecessary prescription, if they know that you demanded one the last ten times.

Second opinions are fine. You may have a serious concern that has not been addressed. You may have worries that are not obvious to the provider. Perhaps you are getting pressure from your extended family to see a specialist. Or maybe you just can't sleep at night. These are all good reasons to get a specialist's input. A good primary care provider understands, and is not defensive about your need to see someone else. She also knows that nine times out of ten, the specialist confirms the primary care provider's opinion, and you leave reassured, and with strengthened confidence in your pediatric office. If this is not the case, or you find yourself asking for outside opinions regularly, there may not be a good fit between you and your provider.

There is probably more worth saying about this topic, but it will have to wait. I have to go update *the list*.

Kidding.

c. Surgeons, legroom and bedside manner

I once sat next to a pilot on a train. He was from Australia and flew for the airline *Qantas*, which has an incredible record for safety. I asked him with whom he would fly, if he ever went somewhere that *Qantas* did not serve. I expected his choices to involve legroom, in-flight meals and friendliness, but instead he started explaining takeoff speeds and other technical factors, which made the planes safer. At this point, it became clear that he was rating airlines the way that I rate doctors.

Ask yourself what you need out of your care provider. Sometimes, it is a good bedside manner and a kind ear. This may be especially true for a primary care or a mental health provider. With specialists, especially surgeons, bedside manner is overrated. Good technical skill and surgical judgment, however, can make the difference between life and death, or at least between a good and a bad outcome.

One of my good surgeon friends used to joke that his initials were G-O-D. Unfortunately, some doctors act as though this were true. But, if their skills are good enough, I will still send them patients. I have been known to prep families about what to expect before sending them to certain arrogant surgeons, especially if the child has a rare condition that few people know how to fix. Most families are happy to see this person, because ultimately what matters is their child's health. In fact, they often thank me both for the head's up and for referring to the best surgeon.

The problem for parents is that you do not know about surgical skill any more than I know about takeoff and landing. Most of us end up making decisions based on what we know, whether it is the in-flight meal or the doctor's friendliness. It sometimes helps to have input from others. Word of mouth, or these days, online ratings are like computers, in general- garbage in, garbage out. Some states and insurance companies publish their own ratings about the performance of doctors and hospitals. Even these are notorious for errors because outcomes depend on the severity of illness. As you would expect, more complex patients and procedures have worse outcomes than straightforward ones, but some doctors and hospitals document severity better than others.

The opinion of someone you trust can still be invaluable. Your primary care provider can often serve this role, as I mentioned above. It is fair game to ask if you would feel comfortable if this surgeon was operating on your child. In fact, this can often lead your doctor to take off her work *hat* for a minute, and really think through a decision. If you do not have this kind of relationship with a primary care provider, there are other tricks. When my Dad needed a cardiologist where he lived, I called the local emergency room to see whom the nurses liked.

Most surgeries go smoothly, just like most plane trips. But when turbulence hits, you want the right Captain to get you through it safely.

d. Sometimes you need a guilt visit to the doctor

With apologies to my own children, sometimes when the pediatrician makes a parenting gaff, he ends up a better doctor.

Andrew was 5 months old. We were at the beach, while on vacation in Nova Scotia. He fell asleep and we laid him in his car seat, but did not buckle him up for fear that he would wake. He stayed asleep until I was carrying him off the beach, at which time he lurched forward and fell face first onto a boardwalk. His poor little face was bruised like he had been in a fight, but thankfully he was otherwise fine.

Me…. Not so much. Let's just say that, 17 years later, I remember it like it was yesterday. Being that we were away, I had none of my medical tools with which to examine him. More importantly, I needed someone to tell me that I was not a bad parent. Off to the local emergency room we went. Andrew charmed all the nurses with his smiling, bruised face. As he clearly was all right, and as the staff reassured us, Sandee and I gradually relaxed and forgave ourselves.

This episode taught me the meaning of the *guilt* visit. As a physician, I knew that many times, a family's presenting medical complaint is just an excuse to ask about something else- this happens most often as the doctor is just about to leave the room. In our case, we were clearly there to confess our sins and ask forgiveness. Rather than make us feel any worse as parents, the staff asked me if I wanted a job at the hospital. I guess they wouldn't do that for a delinquent parent, so what happened couldn't have been too bad!

Some people are born humble; others have humility thrust upon them. Sandee is the former; I am the latter. As with many new graduates, I was occasionally guilty of *doctor knows best*. This changed, in part, after a couple of instances when the parent actually knew better. Still, there is nothing like a *parent of the year* experience to teach how fleeting good health can be, and how none of us are immune to parenting errors. The end result is that I never tell anyone whose child has been hurt, "You need to be careful." If watching your most precious possession in pain has not taught you this, words from me will certainly not matter. Instead, I find myself sharing my own stories of parental inadequacy. And there are many.

It's a funny thing. People seem to really like knowing that doctors screw up as parents, too. While that still reinforces my own parental guilt a little, it is worth it if the family leaves ready to take on their next challenge.

After all, I did drop Andrew on his face.

Chapter 15: Surviving Parenthood

a. X's and Y's of parenting

Stereotypes are like rules- they are made to be broken. Our society has progressed from a one-size-fits-all model, to one that is more flexible and suited to the couple. Whether your relationship is stereotypical or novel, there will still be differences in how you and you partner approach parenting. We can all become better parents by trying to understand our partner's point of view.

As you may know, chromosomes store most of the genetic material in our cells. Although both men and women have 46 chromosomes per cell, women have two of chromosome X, while men have one X and one Y. Now, the first thing that becomes apparent is that it takes more ink to make an X than a Y, and this translates into more genetic material in the female cell than the male. For women, you may think that this explains a lot. Men might counter that we are just simplifying.

An example: Sandee and I usually have our first good conversation of the day just before bed. We will often try to solve the day's problems, or dilemmas, as Sandee likes to call them. She will usually explain the dilemma and ask my opinion, which I will briefly offer. Shortly thereafter, I will be done for the night, and she will again ask my opinion. I will say essentially exactly what I did the first time. By the fourth time round at this conversation, we will often start to become annoyed with each other. She is upset at my lack of depth of conversation, while I insist on only having one opinion, which was offered the first time she asked. I cannot analyze a problem sideways, upside-down, and backwards like she can. In the morning, she calls her best friend and they sort it out.

The approach to problem solving is just one of the ways that we parent differently. In fact, even problem solving itself is a more typical male approach. Many men are more goal-oriented; we want to fix things. Women tend to be more concerned with the process. Again, my own shortcomings can explain it best. When our children were young, Sandee was home most days during the week. She handled things extremely well, but did have the occasional bad day, of course. On one of these days, I was trying to dissect just where the wheels had fallen off. Unable to figure it out, I (stupidly) said, "You know, what the kids are doing is normal." Her reply was fantastic. "I know it's normal! That doesn't mean I like it!" It was at this moment that I realized, very belatedly, that she did not need or want me to solve her day. What she needed was for me to say, "I'm sorry you had a bad day", and to mean it.

Some of you will probably be reading this and thinking, "Well, thank you, Captain Obvious." And you would be right. Many of you are much more emotionally intuitive than me. Still, I am a pediatrician, with a good sense of empathy, so that has to make me more sensitive than most guys. The point is that your partner may also be in need of Captain Obvious at times.

The world is sometimes forgiving to parents who are trying hard. Imagine a trip to the local children's museum with your child. You realize that you have forgotten the diaper bag at just the wrong, smelly time. Desperate, you ask another museum patron if you can borrow a diaper and some wipes. If you are fortunate, you will likely be shown pity. Some other parents will even say, "Aren't you a good to bring her to the museum" (true story, by the way). In the same situation, a different patron might say to a friend, "Can you believe that mother came to the museum and didn't even have a diaper bag?" Unfortunately, women often seem to get a harder time.

Same sex parents have to deal with differing styles, too. Clearly, this presents unique opportunities for changes in role. On the whole, however, parenting with a same sex partner shares many more similarities than differences with those of the opposite sex. I recently heard a gay man advising straight couples about dating etiquette. His advice was very applicable to parenthood. Whoever gets to the door first should open it. Whoever makes the invitation should pay for the meal. If you notice something that your date likes, do that. In a nutshell, be considerate and understanding of your partner.

Some people were born to parent; for others, each day is work. If you are not a natural, you will likely feel insecure, regardless of your gender. The sooner you forgive yourself, the better off you will be. Think of a kid who is a star athlete, versus one who is not, but works her butt off. Ask the coach who she loves having on the team. Nine times out of ten it is the hard worker, and your child will feel the same way about you. Kids understand when you care, and that is what matters. Like so many other things, if you do your best, you can look in the mirror at the end of the day and feel proud.

Doing your best also means understanding your partner, and forgiving him when he fails at a task that you would find easy. Because we are all naturals at some things, and dunces at others.

b.   Children as relationship builders

It's 7 o'clock at night, and the day is winding down. If you have young children, you are probably tired, either because you just cared for the kids all day, or because you were out working, trying to support them. But, as a parent, there is still work to be done. Dinner, dishes, bath and bedtime, or whatever makes up your evening routine. This is a really important time of the day.

It is what pop psychology has come to call *quality time*, the main opportunity during the week for most working families to interact all together. And even though I hate the term itself, I do not underestimate the importance of six to eight pm. A good evening routine can give children an enjoyable and even educational end to their day. Most parents fondly remember the time spent bathing their kids and reading to them, years after that stage has passed. The kids themselves may not remember their earliest days, but many will later talk about bedtime as some of their earliest memories.

What you do during that time is less important than having a consistent routine that works for you. The routine helps the kids know what to expect, and that going to sleep follows. Although exercise or physical play can be a part of it, usually the idea is to help their little engines gradually slow down. If you are musical, it can be a time to sing or play an instrument. The artistic can draw and the imaginative can create stories. It really does not matter, as long as it is enjoyable.

Perhaps most importantly, this may be one of the few times during the week when the entire family can do the same thing at the same time. Much of our time, even in two parent households, is spent tag-teaming at best. One of you watches the kids while the other goes to work. It may be that you both go to work, or that you leave for the evening shift, as she comes home during the day. Regardless, whenever the two of you are both home with the children, you have the chance to parent together. This is a great opportunity in many respects.

Working together lightens the load on everyone. One good approach is, "I'll clear up the dishes. You get the bath running and let me know when it is ready." This way you are efficient, but also saving the fun part- the bath and story time- to do together. Working together on these relatively easy tasks helps prepare you as a parent for the teen years, when the decisions you will make together are often much more difficult. At the point, a united front will help to prevent the kids from playing one against the other.

Some parents struggle with this time of day. It makes me sad to hear a spouse say, "I did bath last night. You do it tonight." This is not to ignore that the evening involves work, or to say that you have to do it together every single night. Noticing that your partner is tired, and offering to do bedtime is a great sign of cooperation. In the same way, asking if it is OK if you take the night off once in a while is a sign that you recognize your own limits. By *asking* your partner, you are showing that you know it is a shared responsibility, and that you would be quite happy to do the same in return another day. On the other hand, if you quarrel regularly over what should be a generally happy time, it may suggest a significant issue for the two of you as a couple.

Kids will learn from what they see. They will learn how a family can work together or against each other. Parents that work well together with young children are likely to co-parent well in later years, even if they have split up as a couple. As we discuss elsewhere, cooperating as parents is the most important factor in determining a child of divorce's emotional health.

Take the time to do things as entire family. Hopefully, you will be having fun. You will also be learning how to work together, setting a good example, and making positive memories for all.

c. My child would never do that

This is possibly the most obnoxious thing that a person can say to a new parent. It is negative in so many ways. It says you have a bad child, and that you are a bad parent. It implies that another person is better than you. It is ignorant, both as a statement and in the lack of knowledge that it shows in those who utter it. As Dr. Suess might say, it is obnoxious in the store, it is obnoxious on the floor. It is obnoxious from a stranger, it's obnoxious from a neighbor.

The main reason to raise this subject at all is to reassure you. Should it be said to you, it is the other person's problem, not yours. Most of the time, it is spoken about behaviors that are perfectly normal. Perhaps your three-year-old just threw a major fit in the grocery store. Normal. Perhaps she will not eat her vegetables at your in-laws' house. Normal. Perhaps your two-year-old just hit or bit you. Normal.

People who say things like this usually try to make themselves feel better by belittling someone else. If it is of any consequence to you, it won't work. Sometimes they feel as though they are child behavior experts, but clearly they are not. Anyone with experience will know that God's gift to parenthood could still have a child that misbehaves. As an example, a nurse-friend recently told me that her first two children were angels. She was very proud of herself and says she judged other parents (which I do not believe because she is too nice). Then they had a third, and the third is *that child.* She is not only a better nurse, she is a better parent, because she realizes that some children have the gift of mischief.

And what if you do have *that child?* All children have great qualities and ones that need work. All adults do, too. We are all working on something during the walk of life. For some, it is a pleasant stroll. For most, it has its peaks and valleys. For a select few, it is Mt. Kilimanjaro. It can be climbed, but the effort is tremendous. And only those who have climbed it before you are in a position to give directions.

And, by the way, whoever you are- your child would, too, do that.

d. Take care of your child's mother

Happy wife, happy life makes a lot of sense to me. I was pleased to read a study recently which suggests there is some scientific truth to this statement- happy wives apparently do lead to happy husbands. Having said that, taking care of your child's mother is especially good advice for the mother herself.

Fathers and mothers both depend on happy children for their own happiness. After all, what good parent would be content while knowing that her child was unhappy? At the same time, a child relies on a well-adjusted parent, preferably two, to help him to make a good start in the world. It is a classic *chicken/egg* scenario, but a parent's emotional health is essential for a child's well being.

Society's demands on women are overwhelming. Women are pressured to be as smart and successful as Hilary Clinton, as attractive as Sophia Vergera, and as kind and nurturing as Mother Teresa. The demands of the day can make you feel like you need to drive like Danica Patrick, too! It is no wonder that a mother's own needs can take a back seat to those of her family. This is also not a good idea, for multiple reasons.

First of all, none of us perform well when we are exhausted. We are all better parents when we get enough rest. We are more patient, understanding, nurturing and fun. Surely, these are good qualities that to convey to our kids. Depression and anxiety are more common when fatigued. Along with exhaustion can also come physical ailments. Our ability to safely supervise little children is also affected.

Sometimes, doing too much for others can be a symptom of personal insecurity. Many of us try to over perform when we are new at a role; parenthood is no different. We can definitely over parent our kids, especially if we prevent them from beginning the normal separation process. As one psychiatrist/friend says, "Separation anxiety is a two way street."

Resentment can also develop after always putting yourself last. Sometimes the resentment is directed towards a partner; other times there is no partner to direct it towards. In those cases especially, we may well put that resentment on to our children. On the other hand, when we get away for a little while, our batteries are recharged. We also feel more balance, set a good example for our children's future lifestyles, and look forward to being back in the company of our little ones.

Of course, men need to have the same kind of balance. Unfortunately, more often that not, our balance tends to be in the other direction; that is, not doing enough for our children or their mother. In the most basic form, this is absence. Too many guys see *sperm donor* as their major role in parenthood. Too many children grow up without a good male role model to show them how a man should act. Even worse is the man who is disruptive or abusive in the home.

Lots of guys do step up. I often ask a mother how well the father is treating her. There is nothing better than hearing, "Oh, he is great.

He is so supportive." This bodes very well for how the family will do in the long run. Sometimes, it is the father who does all the giving. Guys in this situation need to heed the same advice as women.

Extended families, friends and babysitters all play important roles in getting a little down time. If finances are an issue, couples can take turns watching each other's kids. The guys can bond over babysitting while for Girls Night Out and vice versa. The time away does not need to be late or rowdy (because the kids will still be up early!). It can simply be going for a walk, a run or to the library. Any healthy release that relaxes you can work.

One of my favorite questions to ask at the office is, "Do you have any life outside of motherhood?" While motherhood is clearly the most important job you can have, a little time off makes it better for everyone.

e. Going it alone

How does she do it? How does he do it?
We have asked ourselves this question many times, seeing a single parent in action.

In my opinion, there is no job more difficult than parenthood. That opinion was formed as a married parent, where my wife admittedly has done a bigger share of the work. When you have a partner, you have help- someone to take over when you are tired, someone in whom you can confide and with whom you can troubleshoot. It is truly hard for me to imagine how single parents do it.

But they do. According to recent data, a single parent raises one third of children. In fact, two thirds of African American kids live with a single parent. In reality, though, the statistics mean nothing when you are doing all the work. Juggling the many commitments of parenthood requires a great deal of skill. Most of us have certain talents, and other shortcomings. Two parent households can divide the labor, and each can do what they find easier, whether it be organizing the child's day, or staying up late when she won't go to sleep. A single parent has to be Jack-of-all-trades.

Some single parents have the benefit of supportive extended families. I had a friend in university who became a single mother at nineteen. The father was nowhere to be found. She lived with her parents, and the grandparents watched her son while she continued her education. Most impressive was the 21–year-old uncle, who took time every day to spend with his nephew, despite his own college studies. That boy did great, thanks in large part to a strong family network.

As we discussed earlier, some parents have families who are less than supportive. Many times a dysfunctional upbringing will repeat itself in a future generation. Occasionally, a parent has to break out on her own in order to make a fresh start. For most of us, though, the only thing worse than family is no family.

Most cities have programs which can help single parents. A good program can be a godsend. As with every other aspect of parenthood, it is important to for a parent to try to ensure that good intentions are supported by the good actions. There are few things more tragic than a single parent who is working his butt off, only to find out that a *helpful* program ended up being a bad influence, or even worse, a source of neglect or abuse. A single parent, however, may not have the luxury of being too choosy.

Children in single parent families often lack good role model for adult relationships. In my opinion, this is underrated. A boy should see the right way for a man to act, and for a man to treat a partner. He should feel the love of a mother. A girl should see how a partner should treat a woman, and experience equality in the home before going out into the world. Is this unrealistic and naïve? Sure, but that does mean that it should not be a goal for our children. We all wish for our children to be successful in life, and where better to begin than in relationships?

That being said, there are definitely times when going it alone is preferable. As I have said before, a parent who flits in and out a child's life undependably plays mind games with the child. This is never a good thing. A parent who is chemically impaired is better off absent until recovery can be achieved. An abusive parent is better to stay absent. Unfortunately, abusive parents almost always stay that way (unless past substance abuse was the main issue). Leaving a difficult relationship can be the second most difficult thing that a person can do. We have already discussed how complicated the issues can be when trying to leave. However, the only thing more difficult is staying.

It is also not unusual for strong couples to have to endure separation. Our country's recent military history has fragmented families, while a mother or a father serves overseas. This obviously has it's own set of worries. A parent who is killed in service defies adequate words. Those who return often are changed dramatically. Sometimes separation comes after the return from war. These are all tragedies, as is a death due to cancer or other disease. Thankfully, these situations engender a response from the community, and a large show of support. A death due to mental illness or other stigmatized situation will often increase the isolation of a surviving family.

Finally, I should mention the person who is a single parent by choice. Overall, single parenthood rates are increasing. Single parenthood by choice is very difficult to determine since the popularity of marriage varies. Certainly, the rates vary a lot by demographic group. The statistics do not really matter, if that is the case in your household. Clearly, the reasons to choose single parenthood are as varied as the people who choose it. Some mothers who are single by choice truly want and plan it this way. Others do so because of the individual father, not because of a belief in the lifestyle. Whether the reason, it is always better for a parent to be living life in a way that is a conscious expression of being as happy as possible.

Being by yourself is different than being alone. Being alone is different from being lonely. When you are a single parent, you have the potential for all of the above. The goal is to be as happy as your life situation allows, to recognize the extra work involved, and to be comfortable reaching out to others, for the benefit of you and your child.

f.   Softening the sting of splitting up

The last chapter concerned how the parent copes with being alone. This one is about the children. In a word, the key to how the kids will come out of a parental breakup is cooperation.

To be honest, I have always liked the idea that in the event that of a relationship failure, the children should get the house. After all, do we not always tell them that it is not their fault? Why should a young child have to pack a bag twice each week and schlep back and forth between two households, let alone two towns? OK, so I know that is rarely practical, but I wish it were. Truth be told, kids seem to cope with two homes better than most adults would. It is a testament to their resiliency.

Failing this, we still want to maintain the concept of doing what is best for them. Why is cooperation the key? First of all, it just is. Research shows that this to be the case (1). It is worth considering the reasons for a moment. For starters, cooperating at the time of a separation is very difficult. After all, if the adults were getting along so well, there would not be a separation in the first place. It takes a huge effort, and speaks to putting love for the children over our own personal needs. Ironically, it does also serve the needs of the adults, because we all want our children to do well, and there is often tremendous guilt about the effect that the breakup will have on them. Cooperation also increases consistency. As we discussed in the chapter on behavior, it is easier to follow the rules if you know the rules. Cooperative co-parenting will help achieve this goal.

Failure to cooperate is a bad sign. It usually suggests a high toxicity level in the parents' relationship. It means that one or both parents are so upset with the other that this becomes the focus of the adult's energy. Many times this comes simply from intense dislike. Bitterness from infidelity or other breeches of trust can really challenge the ability to cope, as can plain old heartbreak. Occasionally, a true suspicion that one parent will neglect or abuse a child can lead the other to take extreme steps. As a pediatrician, it can be very difficult to sort through these *he said. she said* issues.

Sometimes we are aware of evidence that will make us take sides; most often we have to inform the parents about what will help children of divorce, and hope the adults can begin to act like adults. A parent who has true fear for his or her child has to do what must be done.

Bad-mouthing is worthy of particular mention. Of course, individuals who break up will have bad things to say about each other. That is the nature of the beast, and an adult needs to express these to move on. It is critically important that these words not be spoken in front of the children, or even worse, to the children. Many parents will try to make friends out of, or gain favor from, their children in this way. It is a bad idea. As someone taught me many years ago, no matter how you feel about the other parent, your child is fifty percent that person. You cannot speak ill of the parent without it affecting the child.

Separation and divorce are much more common and generally less stigmatizing than in the past. There are many professionals who can help, from mental health professionals, to teachers. Supportive families can ease the pain. Community services can be utilized. Children need first and foremost to receive love. They need reassurances about their innocence in the cause of the breakup, and they need to know, practically, how their lives will be changed. Focusing your energy in this direction, with the help of resources, can ease the transition.

Last but not least, keep it simple. When giving explanations, imagine you are dealing with a simple topic, like where you are going that day, or what you are going to have for dinner. Be honest, but not so brutally honest as to be scary. Allow time for questions, and do not be surprised if they come much later, at strange moments and times.

If you love them, it will show. And you do, so it will.

g. The death of a child

One of the strange parts of being a pediatrician is that I have been to more funerals for children than I have for adults. This is a dubious distinction, but it has given me a certain window into the hell that awaits grieving parents.

There are so many parents that come into my head at this time, from personal friends, to parents in my practice, to those I have met through my interest in injury prevention. Each has his or her own story, but what they share is sorrow and pain. As safety advocate and father Alan Brown of Georgia puts it, grieving parents are part of an exclusive club that you would not wish for anyone to join.

There are many ways that parents reach the point of their child's death. Some are sudden and unexpected; others are at the end of a long battle. Unlike older individuals, there is no go *good way to go* for

340

children. The anguish of a sudden, unexpected death is certainly unparalleled, but a comfortable, pain-free death is only minimally better. It would be difficult to tell two such grieving parents apart because either way, it is a tragedy. There is no good way for your child to die.

There are no words that are going to do justice to a grieving parent; certainly not ones that I can offer. I think this probably defies words. The only thing that I can do is share a few tips that seem to have helped a little over the years.

For parents:

1. *Expect to feel like life has lost its meaning.* For most of us, children give life its greatest meaning. When you lose your child, you literally do lose meaning. Facing this reality is necessary.

2. *Do whatever it takes to get you out of bed every day.* There are other reasons to live, most notably other children or family members who love and need you. Leverage these people to keep yourself going. Keep their photos close, and constantly remind yourself of their importance to you, and your importance to them.

3. *Talk.* Talking is hard, but it is usually good. Everyone will be different- some might bond with a group, while others would find it extremely irritating. Some will find help professionally, while others will stumble into a person who understands. Most will find that the best ear has been through grief himself.

4. *Be open to medication,* especially if it helps you to avoid self-medication.

5. *Everyone has a different clock for recovery.* There is no time after which grief should lift. Your body does not care about your job, your obligations or your impatience. It will lift when it is ready, and that is okay. Your partner may be on a totally different clock than you. Knowing that you will get there at some point can really relieve the pressure that you are not there yet. (By the way, within this broad range, my own experience is that five years is average. I only mention this so that you know it is a long time.)

6. *Expect to be angry with your partner and family.* Anyone who has been in a long-term relationship knows that we tend to hold ourselves together in public, and then take it out on those we love. This is especially true if there is any perceived guilt or fault that we feel about ourselves or each other, such as having been the driver of the car, or the one who put off the initial medical appointment Work very hard to avoid alienating yourselves from each other. You need each other and you both hurt.

For others:

1. *Go out of your way to say hello.* Many people are afraid to say the wrong thing, and end up saying nothing at all. This increases the isolation of people who already feel isolated. The elephant in the room is too big to avoid. You do not have to be eloquent; an expression of compassion such as, "It is good to see you. You have been in my prayers", is more than enough. It is generally best to avoid, "How are you?" because the answer is universally awful.

2. *Talk about the deceased child to his parents.* Not only do bereaved parents lose their child, they lose the ability to talk about him like the rest of us. Unfortunately, memories are all that these parents have. If you knew him, tell his parents what you loved about him; if you did not know him, ask what he was like. Ask to see pictures, and listen to the stories that will flow out of the pictures.

3. *Cut them a lot of slack.* It is impossible to explain their pain. A long time in practice in one town has given me some great gifts. Near the top of these gifts is the chance to see people who have worked through the grief of the loss of a child. To be honest, many people go years before I see them smile. Then something wonderful happens, usually a wedding or the birth of a grandchild, and they rise like the Phoenix. It is a remarkable experience, and one which I feel fortunate to share with them.

343

Conclusion

Children keep you young.

I started this book with the thought that children keep you young, but first they make you old. It seems only fair that I should end it with thoughts about how they keep you young. And they do, in so many ways.

Recently, I was having a bad day. Nothing major, I was just tired and cranky. Then a series of small things went wrong. I don't actually remember exactly what those things were, but I do remember a child who made it better. His name is Matthew and he is 4 years old. He usually arrives to the office dressed as a cowboy-hat, jeans, vest, and boots, at a minimum. That would be great enough, but on this particular day, he mixed it up a little. His costume of the day was a red cape, along with a matching red mask. How can you stay grumpy in the face of that?

I could tell a hundred other similar stories- a little girl who identified herself as Princess and her brother as Dragon, a boy who liked to be called Cowboy Bob, and another who insisted he could go to space that day even though he had an ear infection because his G Force Corrector would prevent the pressure build-up from bothering his ears. Some of these encounters have come immediately after a truly bad event, including after my return from a child's death in the emergency room. It is no wonder that pediatricians have the lowest suicide rate among physicians, and I am sure it is not just the type of person who chooses this field. It is the kids who lift you up when you are down.

A parent named Marianne, who is now a close friend, was a wonderful caregiver for her severely disabled and retarded son, Petey. He suffered from birth on, and she and her husband Pete did everything possible to try to give him a little quality of life. Upon Petey's death at age ten, Marianne confided in me that she was told early on that they would learn more from Petey than he would from them, and that this had definitely been the case. I realized then that I had learned more from her than she had from me. Many years later, that continues to be true.

There is a new young boy in my practice with multiple medical problems that were not discovered until after his birth. He is the first child for the father, who is in his forties. The father told me that during the pregnancy, he imagined that the boy would be a *fighter*. The child ended up needing open-heart surgery at one month of age, and has several other long-term medical problems, but he continues to improve. As his dad said, he is definitely a fighter, just not quite in the way that he had originally imagined.

Any time that you feel old, go find a young child. Better still, find several playing together. If you watch them, you will soon find yourself smiling. If you join in with them, you will find yourself instinctively doing and saying things from your own childhood, and the feeling will be exhilarating (you may also find your back hurts the next day.)

In other words, the lessons we learn about children are often the ones we learn from children. The lessons are waiting, if we are willing to look and listen.

###

References

Chapter 1

c.

(1) American Academy Of Pediatrics. (2104) *Caring for Your Baby and Young Child, 6th Edition: Birth to Age 5*. Bantam.

d.

(1) LeDoux, JE.Prog. (2012) Evolution of Human Emotion. A View Through Fear. *Brain Res.* 195: 431–442.

(2) Areias ME, Kumar R, Barros H, and Figueiredo E. (1996) Correlates of postnatal depression in mothers and fathers. *Br J Psychiatry.* Jul;169(1):36-41

e.

(1) Banas JA, Dunbar N, Rodriguez D; Liu S (2011) A Review of Humor in Educational Settings: Four Decades of Research. Communication Education, 60: 1, 115 — 144

(2) Stoeber, J. and Janssen, D.P. (2011). Perfectionism and coping with daily failures: Positive reframing helps achieve satisfaction at the end of the day. *Anxiety, Stress, & Coping,* 24 (5). pp. 477-497

h.

(1) Zimmerman FJ, Christakis DA, Meltzoff AN.(2007) Associations between media viewing and language development in children under age 2 years. *J Pediatr.*151(4):364-8.

k.

(1) Mayer EA, Naliboff B, and Munakata . (2000). The evolving neurobiology of gut feelings. *J Prog Brain Res.* 122:195-206.

Chapter 2

c.

(1) Office for National Statistics licensed under the Open Government Licence v.2.0 (2014) Gestation-specific infant mortality in England and Wales, 2010 http://www.ons.gov.uk/ons/rel/child-health/gestation-specific-infant-mortality-in-england-and-wales/2010/gestation-specific-infant-mortality-in-england-and-wales--2010.html

(2) Stoll BJ, Hansen NI, Bell EF, et al. (2010) Neonatal outcomes of extremely preterm infants from the NICHD Neonatal Research Network. *Pediatrics* 126(3):443-56.

(3) Platt MJ. (2014) Outcomes in preterm infants. *Public Health.* 128(5):399-403.

(4) Behrman RE and Stith Butler A, Editors. (2006) *Preterm Birth: Causes, Consequences, and Prevention.* The National Academies Press. Washington, DC

(5) Iams J.D.(2014) Prevention of Premature Parturition. *N Engl J Med* 370:254-261

(6) Miller, B. (2013, November 22) Ward Miles-First Year. Retrieved from http://www.youtube.com

(7) Howse JL and Katz M. (2013) Conquering Prematurity. *Pediatrics* 131(1): 1 -2

d.

(1) Sirin H, Weiss HB, Sauber-Schatz EK and Dunning K (2007) Seat Belt use, Counseling and Motor-Vehicle Injury During Pregnancy: Results from a Multi-State Population-Based Survey. *Matern Child Health* 11:505–510

(2) Kugelman A and Colin AA. Late Preterm Infants: Near Term But Still in a Critical Developmental Time Period *Pediatrics* 132 (4) 741 -751

(3) Ehrenthal DB1, Jiang X and Strobino DM. (2010) Labor induction and the risk of a cesarean delivery among nulliparous women at term. *Obstet Gynecol* . 116(1):35-42.

e.

(1) Patrick SW, Schumacher RE, Benneyworth BD et al. (2012) Neonatal Abstinence Syndrome and Associated Health Care Expenditures United States, 2000-2009;*JAMA*;307(18):1934-1940.

(2) Behnke M and Smith VC; Committee on Substance Abuse; Committee on Fetus and Newborn.(2013).Prenatal substance abuse: short- and long-term effects on the exposed fetus. *Pediatrics.* 131(3): e1009-24.

Chapter 3

a.

(1) Walton, GE, Bower, NJA and Bower, TGR (1992) Recognition of familiar faces by newborns. *Infant Brain and Development*, 15:265-9.

b.

(1) World Health Organization, (2014, February), Retrieved from: http://www.who.int/mediacentre/factsheets/fs342

(2) American Academy of Pediatrics, Section on Breastfeeding.(2012) Breastfeeding and the use of human milk *Pediatrics.*; 129(3): e827-41.

(3) National Center for Disease Prevention and Health Promotion Breastfeeding report card CDC 2014. Retrieved from http://www.cdc.gov/breastfeeding

c.

(1) *The Common Sense Book of Baby and Child Care* written by Benjamin Spock, first published in 1946.

(2) Conde-Agudelo A, Belizán JM, and Diaz-Rossello J. (2011) Kangaroo mother care to reduce morbidity and mortality in low birthweight infants.. *Cochrane Database Syst Rev.* Mar 16;(3)

(3) Esposito G, Yoshida S and Ohnishi R. (2013) Infant Calming Responses during Maternal Carrying in Humans and Mice. *Current Biology*, 23(9): 739-745,

(4) Zero to Three: National Center for Infants, Toddlers and Families (2014). Taken from: http://www.zerotothree.org/child-development/brain-development/baby-brain-map.html

e.

(1) Junger S. (1997). *The Perfect Storm.* New York, NY. Publisher: W.W Norton

h.

(1). Romanello S, Spiri D and Marcuzzi E (2013). Association between childhood migraine and history of infantile colic. *JAMA* 309(15):1607-12

(2) Fronsdal G (2001) Taken from http://www.insightmeditationcenter.org/books-articles/articles/impermanence

i.

(1) Sedlak TW and Snyder SH. (2004) Bilirubin benefits: cellular protection by a biliverdin reductase antioxidant cycle. *Pediatrics.* 113(6):1776-82

Chapter 4

a.

(1) Lightdale, JR and Gremse DA. (2013) Section on Gatroenterology, Hepatology and Nutrition. Clinical Report Gastroesophageal Reflux: Management Guidance for the Pediatrician., *Pediatrics.* 131(5): e1684 - 1695.

d.

(1) Lack G. Food Allergy (2008) *N Engl J Med*; 359:1252-1260

(2) Food allergy: A practice parameter update-2014.(2014) Sampson HA, Aceves S, Bock SA, *J Allergy Clin Immunol.* pii: S0091-6749(14)00672-1

(3) Huh SY, Rifas-Shiman SL, Taveras EM (2011) Timing of Solid Food Introduction and Risk of Obesity in Preschool-Aged Children *Pediatrics* 127:3 e544-e551

(4) Du Toit G, Roberts G, Sayre PH et al. (2015) *N Eng J Med*. 372(9): 803-13. Randomized Trial of Peanut Consumption in Infants at Risk for Peanut Allergy

(5) Arnon SS, Midura TF, Damus K, et al. (1979). Honey and other environmental risk factors for infant botulism. *J Pediatr* 94(2): 331-6

i.

(1) Mayo Clinic Staff. (2014) Taken from http://www.mayoclinic.org/healthy-living/nutrition-and-healthy-eating/in-depth/fat/art-20045550

(2) Vannice G and Rasmussen H (2014) Position of the academy of nutrition and dietetics: dietary fatty acids for healthy adults *Acad Nutr Diet.* 114(1): 136-53.

(3) Ogata BN and Hayes D, (2014). Position of the Academy of Nutrition and Dietetics: nutrition guidance for healthy children ages 2 to 11 years *J Acad Nutr Diet.* 114(8): 1257-76.

j.

(1) Nutritional info for Mott's 100% Apple Juice. 2014. Taken from http://www.motts.com/products/2/100-apple-juice

(2) Nutritional info for JuicyJuice 100% Apple Juice. 2014Taken from http://www.juicyjuice.com/Products/Juicy-Juice-Fruit-Juice/Apple.aspx

k.

(1) Gray J (1992) *Men are from Mars, Women are from Venus.* Ne York, NY. Harper Collins

(2) Choby BA, George S (2008) Toilet training. *Am Fam Physician.*1;78(9):1059-64.

Chapter 5

a.

(1) United Nations Children's Fund (2013) *The State of the World's Children.* New York, NY.

(2) Moon C, Lagercrantz H and Kuhl PK. (2013) Language experienced in utero affects vowel perception after birth: a two-country study. *Acta pediatrica* 102:156–160

b.

(1) The Magic School House. (1994-98). Public Broadcasting Corporation.

Chapter 6

a.

(1) Moon RY. Task Force on Sudden Infant Death Syndrome. (2011) SIDS and Other Sleep-Related Infant Deaths: Expansion of Recommendations for a Safe Infant Sleeping Environment. *Pediatrics.* 128(5): e1341–67

(2) Semple A.(2008) What influences baby-sleeping behaviour at night: A review of evidence. *New Digest.*

d.

(1) Thomas W. Phelan (2104) *1-2-3 Magic: Effective Discipline for Children 2-12* Parentmagic, Inc.; Glen Ellyn, IL.

e.

(1) Orr B (2013) *Orr: My Story.* GP Putnum's Sons. New York, NY.

f.

(1) Dr. Suess (1990) Oh, The Places You'll Go! Random House. New York, NY.

h.

(1) Steiner H, Remsing L and the Work Group on Quality Issues. (2007) Practice parameter for the assessment and treatment of children and adolescents with oppositional defiant disorder. *J Am Acad Child Adolesc Psychiatry.* 46(1): 126-41

(2) American Academy of Child and Adolescent Psychiatry.(2013) *ODD: A Guide for Families.* Taken from: http://www.aacap.org

(3) Greene RW. (2014) *The Explosive Child: A New Approach for Understanding and Parenting Easily Frustrated, Chronically Inflexible Children. 5 Rev Upd edition* Harper Paperbacks; New York, NY

i.

(1) Miriam-Webster Dictionary (2014). Taken from http://www.merriam-webster.com

(2) Wiseman R. (2003) *Queen Bees and Wannabes: Helping Your Daughter Survive Cliques, Gossip, Boyfriends, and Other Realities of Adolescence Paperback –* : Three Rivers Press; New York, NY

j.

(1) Kirkorian HL, Wartella EA and Anderson DR.(2008) Media and young children's learning. *Future Child.* 18(1): 39-61.

(2) Lapierre MA, Taylor Piotrowski J and Linebarger DL. (2012) Background Television in the Homes of US Children. *Pediatrics* 130(5): 839-846

(3) Brown A, (2011) Council on Communications and Media. Media Use by Children Younger Than 2 Years Council on Communications and Media. *Pediatrics.* 128(5): 1040-5.

(4) Brito N, Barr R, McIntyre P, et al J. (2012) Long-term Transfer of Learning from Books and Videos during Toddlerhood *Exp Child Psychol.* 111(1): 108-19.

(5) Chonchaiya W and Pruksananonda C. (2008) Television viewing associates with delayed language development. *Acta Paediatr.* 97(7): 977-82

(6) Zimmerman FJ, Christakis DA and Meltzoff AN. (2007) Associations between media viewing and language development in children under age 2 years. *J Pediatr* 151(4): 364-8

(7) Christakis DA, Gilkerson J, Richards JA, et al. (2009) Audible television and decreased adult words, infant vocalizations, and conversational turns: a population-based study. *Arch Pediatr Adolesc Med.* 163(6): 554-8

Chapter 7

b.

(1) Stibich AS , Yagan M and Sharma V (2000) Cost-effective post-exposure prevention of poison ivy dermatitis. *Int J Dermatol.* 39(7): 51.

c.

(1) Paller AS, Hawk JLS, Honig P et al. (2011) New Insights About Infant and Toddler Skin: Implications for Sun Protection P. *Pediatrics* 128(1): 92 -102

d.

(1) American Academy of Pediatrics.(2012) *Red Book Report of the Committee on Infectious Disease, 29th Edition.* Elk Grove Village, IL

(2) Center for Disease Control (2014). Taken from :
http://www.cdc.gov/parasites/bedbugs/faqs.html
(3) Center for Disease Control (2104) . Taken from:
http://www.cdc.gov/parasites/scabies/health_professionals/meds.html
f.
(1) Center for Disease Control. (2014) Taken from:
http://www.cdc.gov/sids

Chapter 8

a.
(1) US Department of Health and Human Services (2014). Taken from:
http://www.vaccines.gov/basics/effectiveness
(2) Immunization Action Coalition (2014). Taken from:
http://www.immunize.org/askexperts
b.
(1) Wikipedia. (2014) Taken from
http://en.wikipedia.org/wiki/Ignaz_Semmelweiss
(2) Jefferson T1, Del Mar CB (2011) Physical interventions to interrupt
or reduce the spread of respiratory viruses. *Cochrane Database Syst Rev.*
6;(7).
f.
(1) Showerman G. (1914) *The Microphobiac* From The Unpopular Review
Princeton Vol 1. New York Henry Holt and Co.

Chapter 9

c.
(1) Geggel R, Horowitz LM, Brown EA, et al.(2002) Parental anxiety
associated with referral of a child to a pediatric cardiologist for evaluation
of a Still's murmur. *J Pediatr.* 140(6):747.

Chapter 10

a.
(1) J Ramos-Jorge, I. Pordeus, ML. Ramos-Jorge, et al (2011) Prospective
Longitudinal Study of Signs and Symptoms Associated With Primary
Tooth Eruption. *Pediatrics* 128(3): 471 -47.

Chapter 11

a.

(1) Durbin DR Committee on Injury, Poisoning and Violence Prevention. (2011) Policy Statement––Child Passenger Safety *Pediatrics* 127(4): 788-93.

b.

(1) Center for Disease Prevention and Control (September 26, 2014) Taken from: http://www.cdc.gov/MotorVehicleSafety

d.

(1) Suellen M Walker (2014) Neonatal pain. *Paediatr Anaesth* 24(1): 39–48
(2) Kuppermann N1, Holmes JF, Dayan PS et al.(2009) Identification of children at very low risk of clinically-important brain injuries after head trauma: a prospective cohort study. *Lancet.* 374(9696): 1160-70.

e.

(1) Young Guns: A Diane Sawyer Special. (2014). Taken from: http://abc.go.com/shows/2020/
(2) Dowd MD, Sege RD Council on Injury, Violence, and Poison Prevention Executive Committee; American Academy of Pediatrics. (2012) Policy Statement: Firearm-Related Injuries Affecting the Pediatric Population *Pediatrics.* 130(5): e1416-23

Chapter 12

e.

(1) Regina M Milteer, Ginsburg KR (2012) The Importance of Play in Promoting Healthy Child Development and Maintaining Strong Parent-Child Bond: Focus on Children in Poverty. *Pediatrics.* 129(1): e204-13.
(2) Chaucer G. (2008) *The Cantebury Tales.* Oxford World's Classics. Oxford University Press Oxford, UK.

f.

(1) Strasburger VC1, Jordan AB, Donnerstein E. (2010) Health effects of media on children and adolescents. *Pediatrics.* 125(4): 756-67.
(2) McLuhan M (1964) *Understanding Media: The Extensions of Man.* MIT Press. Cambridge, MA

Chapter 13

a.

(1) Zimmeran GL, Olsen CG and Bosworth MF A 'Stages of Change' Approach to Helping Patients Change Behavior (2000) *Am Fam Physician* 1;61(5):1409-1416.

(2) O'Connor RJ. (2012) Non-cigarette tobacco products: What have we learned and where are we headed? *Tob Control.* 21(2): 181–190

c.

(1) Center for Disease Control and Prevention (2014). Taken from: http://www.cdc.gov/violenceprevention

(2) Wilkins, N, Tsao, B , Hetz,M et al (2014) Connecting the Dots: An Overview of the Links Among Multiple Forms of Violence. Center for Disease Control Institute.

Chapter 15

e.

(1) US Department of Commerce (2011) Social and Economic Characteristics of Currently Unmarried Women with a recent birth: 2011. Taken from: www.census.gov

(2) Kids Count Data Center (2014). Taken from: http://datacenter.kidscount.org/

f. (1) American Academy of Child and Adolescent Psychiatry (2014). Taken from: http://www.aacap.org

Acknowledgements

This book could not be written without the help of many people. For their review of the manuscript, I would like to sincerely thank Catherine Parkinson, Taryn Carlson-Andrews, Margaret and Lloyd Gillis, Dorothy and Edward Parkinson, and Kate Thomas, Drs. Jonathan Davis, Paul DeMeo, Frank Emerling,, Lois Lee, Emily O'Connell, Garrett Zella,

For allowing me to use the cover photo of their beautiful daughter Paige, I thank Geody and Kirsten Moore.

Finally, I am thankful for all the teachers that have instructed me over the years. The most important of these have been children, including my own- Catherine, Andrew and Christopher, as well as my very patient wife, Sandee.

Subject Index

About the author

Greg Parkinson grew up and attended medical school in Canada. In 1995, he began full-time practice at Falmouth Pediatric Associates in Cape Cod, Massachusetts. He is the Chair of Injury, Violence and Poison Prevention for the Massachusetts Chapter of the American Academy of Pediatrics, and has received awards from the National Highway Traffic Safety Administration, the Commonwealth of Massachusetts, the Massachusetts Medical Society, and the Massachusetts Intercollegiate Athletic Association. He lives with his wife, Sandee, and three children, ages 15-20.

Made in the USA
Middletown, DE
16 October 2015